HOMEOPATHIC FAMILIES

20 remedies coming alive

vienna study group

initiated by Massimo Mangialavori

D1726206

2003

Authors of the vienna study group:

Ruth v. Bonin-Schulmeister
Ursula Kogler
Uta Santos-König
Doris Heu
Peter Bondes
Wolfgang Reitinger
Ulli Wessely
Renate Kastner

Copyright: with the authors
Produced by Books on Demand GmbH, Norderstedt, Germany
Wien 2003
ISBN 3-8330-0239-5

CONTENTS

INTRODUCTION

I don´t serve you the cooked fish, I want to teach you fishing...

This was an often-used sentence of M. Mangialavori when the enthusiasm in our study group (especially after lunch) went low and we expected another fascinating case presentation of a not so well known remedy.

The aim of this study group in Vienna between 1999 and 2002 was not only to learn about "small remedies" but even more to find a methodological approach to study new remedies, and to work on them in a group of homoeopaths. But how to fish for remedies as Citrus vulgaris, Sphingurus, Pulex, Yohimbe? We always started from a polychrest, trying to find themes that are fundamental for a good prescription of this remedy. This polychrest standing in the centre of a so-called family is giving the fundamental themes for the other "small remedy" members of this family.

The members of our study group collected all the available information about the exotic sounding remedies, and in presenting the facts and discussing them in our group with the guidance of M. Mangialavori the themes of a family emerged. M. Mangialavoris cases of these lesser-known remedies presented in our study group together with the collected facts made it understandable what is fundamental for a family and how the same theme is varied within a family.

This book gives you an idea what remedy to think of when your really good prescription of Silica was not successful. Have you ever thought of Bambusa, Equisetum, Sphingurus ...? They all belong to the Silica family. Here you get the information what themes you will have to find in your patient, to think of a certain family of remedies. This book takes you on a journey to a new approach of remedies in thinking of families and themes.

We hope that in reading it, you take part in the fascinating process of remedies that come alive when a group of people is working together and something beyond the mere facts starts to reveal.

ABOUT THE BOOK

Every case presented in this book comes from a patient of M. Mangialavori. They all have a follow up of at least two years in which period they were treated exclusively with the one remedy mentioned.

The intensity of description of each group of remedies varies according to the development of the method over the years and the different ways of elaborating the information by different authors. We tried as well as possible to keep to a consequent structure and layout through the chapters to understand quickly the importance of a theme for a certain remedy.

A key for the presentation of themes is used in this book, which is the same as used in M. Mangialavori's program Tesi:

Themes of remedies

Bold = fundamental theme, a requirement to prescribe this remedy.
Underlined = important theme, to observe in the majority of cases.
Plain type = a theme that can be observed often, but is not so important.
CAPITALS (whether bold or underlined or plain) = differentiation within a family. A theme that differentiates this special remedy from the others in the same family.
Description of the substance, its use and all available information

The index shows all remedies mentioned in a seminary that were not the main subject and came into differential diagnosis. In the text one finds them as *Differentiation.*

SILICA - LIKE REMEDIES

When studying this subject you see how abundant this element is on our planet, especially in our European area. So this substance is absolutely important.
When talking about Silica, we do not mean just one remedy but a class of remedies including not only Silica terra and Silica marina but also several salts like Calcarea-silicata, Alumina-silicata or Kalium-silicatum and others.

We can consider elements as dynamic processes. Silica represents a big process, like Natrum, Calcarea or Magnesia. It is not just a polychrest, it is a manifestation of a way of adaptation, of a way of relating to the environment, and this does not only concern Silica, but also a huge class of remedies of which Silica is probably the best known. Our task is to try to understand the most important themes, the most important characteristics of this Silica-process that we will also find in other remedies We consider these remedies close to Silica and therefore belonging to the Silica-family. So we are working on something quite well known and on something not at all known. Equisetum e.g. is one of the not so well known remedies in homeopathy even if we have some information about it. When we compare the homeopathic information with the one we have from our herbalist tradition, especially in our area, we can see that equisetum as a plant is used a lot. It is a polychrest in herbalist medicine and probably we do not use it as often as we could in homeopathy.

On the other side Bambusa is a big remedy and it is known from one of the few very well done recent provings. Bambusa has not only a big amount of symptoms, it was a very good choice for proving because bamboo is a plant with a lot of symbolism, a plant which has been traditionally used in our planet, not only as a medicine, but for many other purposes. Therefore in the next years Bambusa will probably be a real polychrest. One of the differences between Bambusa and Equisetum is the far bigger symbolical importance of bamboo. Then there is Sphingurus. It is practically unknown in terms of homeopathy. There are some strange stories about this animal, and there are many animals close to the porcupine that are not well known at all. M. Mangialavori has some very good cases of Sphingurus so that from these cured cases some ideas will arise about this group of animals. It is interesting that the quills of the porcupine have an appearance close to that of equisetum. They are yellow or white and brown in stripes and resemble the knots of equisetum and bamboo. The porcupine is one of the very few ancient animals coming from the world of rodents. Very recently the proving of the milk of the rat and mouse and hamster was done, so you can get some more homeopathic information about these animals. M. Mangialavori considers the remedies Hekla lava, Lac felinum and Castor equi close to Silica, which is from the point of view of the substance also very close to Sphingurus. Castor equi is the former thumb of the horse, a rudiment from a time when horses used to walk on three toes. The horse now walks on one finger. The thumb rudiment is situated on the inner side of the leg, a thickened part of the skin, which is exfoliated spontaneously when cleaning the hoof of the horse. It contains some silica and is a similar material to the spine of the porcupine. It is a tissue similar to the human nail.

Obviously there are other ideas and other remedies close to Silica that are not discussed now because there is not yet enough evidence. Including the above-mentioned remedies into the Silica-group means that M. Mangialavori has at least three or four cured cases of each of them. So returning to the idea of Silica as a process, as an archetype of a certain dynamic, it is a specific, quite widespread way of reacting of our system. We will try to define what is important in this process, what are the themes common to all the members of the Silica-group and what are the characteristics of each member of this family – specifically also for Silica itself.

SILICA

Descriptions:

The element Silica:
Chemical symbol: Si
Atomic weight: 28,086
Atomic number: 14

Density: 2,33g/cm3
Melting point: 1414°C
Boiling point: 3265°C
Si is grey and brittle.

The Latin name is Silex, in German called Kieselstein. It was found very late. Silica was prepared by reduction of tetra fluid and Kalium. The pure substance of silica is quite difficult to extract. In the periodic table it is one of the main element of the carbon group.

One quarter of the earth's soil is made up of silica. You find a lot of silica in the stone meteorites; also the moon and the mars contain lots of silica, whereas in the sun, which contains lots of helium and hydrogen, you only find 0,002 %.

Quartz

A colourless or toned crystal, is the main form of silica. You can find many different forms as: achat, amethyst, citrin, jaspis, onyx, opal, topaz, tiger-eye. Since ancient times they were used as jewels. Nearly all the half precious stones contain silica. Raw silica is produced in Norway and Brazil, recently also China and Venezuela. Quartz is a widely spread mineral of many varieties that consists primarily of silica, or silicon dioxide ($SiO2$). Minor impurities such as lithium, sodium, potassium, and titanium may be present. Quartz has attracted attention since the earliest times; water-clear crystals were known to the ancient Greeks as krystallos - hence the name crystal, or more commonly rock crystal. Quartz is the second mineral in the Earth's crust after feldspar. It occurs in nearly all acid igneous, metamorphic and sedimentary rocks. It is an essential mineral in such silica-rich rocks as granites, granodiorites and rhyolites. It is highly resistant to weathering and tends to concentrate in sandstones and other detrital rocks. Secondary quartz serves as cement in sedimentary rocks of this kind, forming overgrowths on detrital grains. Microcrystalline varieties of silica known as chert, flint, agate, and jasper consist of a fine network of quartz. Metamorphism of quartz-bearing igneous and sedimentary rocks typically in-creases the amount of quartz and its grain size.

Quartz exists in two forms: (1) alpha-, or low, quartz, which is stable up to 573° C (1,063° F), and (2) beta-, or high, quartz, stable above 573° C. The two are closely related, with only small movements of their constituent atoms during the alpha-beta transition. The structure of beta-quartz is hexagonal, with either a left- or right-handed symmetry group equally populated in crystals. The structure of alpha-quartz is trigonal, again with either a right- or left-handed symmetry group. At the transition temperature the tetrahedral framework of beta-quartz twists, resulting in the symmetry of alpha-quartz; atoms move from special space group positions to more general positions. At temperatures above 867° C (1,593° F), beta-quartz changes into tridymite, but the transformation is very slow because bond breaking takes place to form a more open structure. At very high pressures alpha-quartz transforms into coesite (q.v.) and at still higher pressures, stishovite (q.v.). Such phases have been observed in impact craters.

Quartz is piezoelectric: a crystal develops positive and negative charges on alternate prism edges when it is subjected to pressure or tension. The charges are proportional to the change in pressure. Because of its piezoelectric property, a quartz plate can be used as a pressure gauge, as in depth-sounding apparatus. Just as compression and tension produce opposite charges, the converse effect is that alternating opposite charges will cause alternating expansion and contraction. A section cut from a quartz crystal with definite orientation and dimensions has a natural frequency of this expansion and contraction (i.e., vibration) that is very high, measured in millions of vibrations per second. Properly cut plates of quartz are used for frequency control in radios, televisions, and other electronic communications equipment and for crystal-controlled clocks and watches. Any one of the forms of silicon dioxide ($SiO2$), including quartz, tridymite, cristobalite, coesite, stishovite, melanophlogite, lechatelierite, and chalcedony.

Various kinds of silica minerals have been produced synthetically, among which are keatite and silicalite. Except for stishovite, all silica minerals are made up of tetrahedral groups comprised of four oxygen atoms surrounding a central silicon. Each tetrahedral group shares an oxygen atom with another tetrahedral group, forming a three-dimensional structure. The principal difference among the various silica minerals is the detailed geometry of the arrangement of tetrahedra, which gives rise to different crystal structures and thus physical properties. Quartz has a relatively dense packing of tetrahedra compared to tridymite and cristobalite, which exhibit relatively large open cavities. This packing difference is reflected in their densities: 2.65, 2.32, 2.26 grams per cubic centimetre for quartz, cristobalite, and tridymite, respectively. Each of these three polymorphs of silica has a field of stability under equilibrium conditions, but because transformation from one structure to another is sluggish, tridymite and cristobalite are found within the stability field of quartz. Each of the polymorphs also has high- and low-temperature modifications that are only slightly different structurally. Therefore, under low-pressure conditions, low-quartz is stable until 573° C (1,063° F), at which point high-quartz becomes stable. At 867° C (1,593° F), high-quartz transforms to tridymite. The high-low transformations require only slight displacements of the tetrahedral groups and occur rapidly. Compositionally, quartz is usually quite pure, with only traces of other elements. In contrast, tridymite and cristobalite may contain up to about one percent by weight of impurities because of the open nature of their framework, which easily accommodates other atoms, especially those of aluminium, sodium, potassium, and lithium.

Quartz is the second most abundant mineral in the Earth's crust and is present in many igneous rocks (e.g., granite and syenite) and in hydrothermal vein deposits. Because it is both chemically and mechanically stable at low temperature, quartz persists in clastic sedimentary rocks. Tridymite and cristobalite occur in volcanic rocks such as rhyolite and slowly invert to quartz polymorphs. Of the other silica phases, coesite and stishovite are high-pressure polymorphs found where quartz was shocked by meteorite impact. Coesite also occurs in some eclogite xenoliths from the Earth's upper mantle. Stishovite is unlike other silica phases in that silicon is in octahedral rather than tetrahedral coordination, resulting in a high density of 4.3 g/cc. Keatite is a high-pressure polymorph, but it has not been found in nature. Chalcedony is cryptocrystalline silica consisting of minute quartz crystals and sub microscopic pores. Melanophlogite has an open structure large enough to occlude sulfur species. Lechatelierite is silica glass (amorphous) and is only rarely found in nature.

Traditional use

Silica together with quartzite and firestone is one of the first materials used by man to produce tools and weapons.

Technical use

Quartz has great economic importance. Many varieties are gemstones, including amethyst, citrine, smoky quartz, and rose quartz. Sandstone, composed mainly of quartz, is an important building stone. Large amounts of quartz sand (also known as silica sand) are used in the manufacture of glass and ceramics and for foundry moulds in metal casting. Crushed quartz is used as an abrasive in sandpaper, silica sand is employed in sandblasting, and sandstone is still used whole to make whetstones, millstones, and grindstones. Silica glass (also called fused quartz) is used in optics to transmit ultraviolet light. Tubing and various vessels of fused quartz have important laboratory applications, and quartz fibres are employed in extremely sensitive weighing devices. Silica and its compounds are of enormous technical use in so many different fields as ceramic, glass, cement etc. Silicon – being a synthetic organic polymer of silica is used for denture and artificial limbs.

Because of the above mentioned piezoelectric effect there are lots of possibilities for electronically use: Silicon is the material most often used in diodes, transistors, integrated circuits, microprocessors, RAM and ROM memory, detectors and infra-red lenses, light emitting diodes (LEDs), photographic developers, solar cells, charged coupled devices (CCDs, used in portable television cameras), thyristors for power circuits, and other devices. You can get some idea of how important it is quantitatively speaking when you think that more than 98% of all the devices containing semiconductors that are made in the world use silicon as the basic material.

Semiconductors

In the 1950s, the most commonly used semiconductor material was germanium. This was subsequently replaced by silicon because it was frequently unusable, due to the severe loss of current at the connection. Among the other advantages of silicon are an energy gap of 1.1eV (Germanium has 0.8) and the capacity to resist temperatures up to 150°C, compared with 100°C for germanium. With the advent of planar technology, the practical success of silicon was assured. In particular, the excellent quality of silicon oxide grown thermally as an isolator in MOS (metal-oxide-semiconductors) integrated circuits was responsible for a rapid development in miniaturisation and the exponential leap in the number of components in integrated circuits. The resistance of intrinsic silicon (not doped) is about 2,300,000 ohms/cm (in intrinsic germanium it is about 40 ohms/cm). This allows rectifying devices with a high breaking strain to be obtained. Silicon, moreover, costs about ten times less than germanium.

The crystalline structure of silica is the best known and most widely used silicon element. Each atom of silica shares its four-valent electrons with the four atoms adjacent to it. This leads to the creation of zones with a relatively high electronic density (two valent electrons for every zone). These link all the atoms of the crystal together and form the so-called covalent bonds. The crystalline structure can be represented by a bi-dimensional model in which the rings stand for the silica atoms without their four-valent electrons, which therefore contain a positive electrical charge equivalent to four times that of the electron. At a temperature of absolute zero, the valent electrons, joined in covalent bonds, cannot receive energy due to the thermal agitation. However, if they do not receive energy from the outside, they cannot leave the zones assigned to them, corresponding to the lowest values of potential energy. At absolute zero, silica (like every other silicon) therefore acts as an isolator. The situation changes at significantly higher temperatures, for example at room temperature. This is because the equilibrium state of the zones that form covalent bonds can be destroyed by the thermal agitation. Indeed, some of the electrons that form the covalent bonds can acquire enough energy to escape from their original zones and move freely, even to other zones in the structure. Some of the covalent bonds can therefore be broken. The destruction of a covalent bond gives rise to two distinct processes. While the electron that has acquired sufficient energy to break the bond moves freely through the crystalline structure, a valent electron involved in another bond with one of the adjacent atoms can repair the broken bond. This electron neutralises an atom that has been temporarily deprived of an electron, but at the same time it leaves behind it a new vacancy for an electron, or a lacuna (i.e., a hole). While the first process is similar to that responsible for the phenomena of conduction in metals, the second represents an electrical movement of a different kind. This has the effect of moving a lacuna from one atom to another. It is clear, therefore, that the destruction of a covalent bond involves the simultaneous liberation of two carriers of charges that are of opposite poles: an electron (a negative carrier) and the lacuna (a positive carrier).

We can consider the importance of the computer in our life at the change of this millennium. Silica is an essential part of all the technology that belongs to electronics. It is an essential part of this development in our culture. For transistors chips only this element was used. It is not by chance that electricity is going just in one direction like the extremes of yes and no we will find in a Silica person.

This yes and no like in silica it is also only in one direction. They started using germanium but it was very expensive and not so good as silica. In the next future they will probably change this element. Silica is not quick enough for further development. The next substance used for this purpose will probably be copper.

Medicine/Pharmacy/Medicine

Silica is an important trace element; a lot of plants are using silica to build up their structure. The cover of rice is very rich with silica as well as different classes of silica containing algae and polygonaceae like buckwheat (Fagopyrum), rhubarb (Rheum), and sorrel (Rumex). Equisetum and Bambusa collect their silica close to the knots.

The human body contains 1,5g of silica, especially in nails and hair. For the growth of bones, cartilage and connective tissue it is indispensable. The substance itself is non-toxic. But the fine dust of quartz can form knots in the connective tissue of the lungs, called silicosis. Thomas Bernhard, an Austrian writer, died of silicosis.

Silicon is necessary for the association between cells, and one or more macromolecules such as osteonectin, which affects cartilage composition and ultimately cartilage calcification.

In spite of the technical adequacy of existing protective equipment, free silica (SiO2), or crystalline quartz, is still a major occupational hazard. In the United States, estimates of potential numbers of exposed workers range between 1.2 and 3 million people. The major occupational exposures include mining, stone-cutting, and employment in abrasive industries, foundry work, packing of silica flour, and quarrying, particularly of granite. Most often, progressive pulmonary fibrosis (silicosis) occurs in a dose-response fashion after many years of exposure. The nodular fibrosis may be progressive in the absence of further exposure, with coalescence and formation of non-segmental conglomerates of irregular masses in excess of 1 cm in diameter. These masses become quite large and are characteristic of PMF. Significant functional impairment with both restrictive and obstructive components may be associated with this form of silicosis. In the late stages of the disease, ventilatory failure may develop. In more subtle cases, CT may be helpful both in identifying nodules, which are preferentially located in the posterior aspect of the upper lobes, as well as in identifying larger opacities and more coalescence than might be noted on regular chest x-rays. Patients with silicosis are at greater risk of acquiring Mycobacterium tuberculosis infections (silicon-tuberculosis) and atypical mycobacterial infections. Because the frequency with which tuberculosis has been found at autopsy in patients with PMF exceeds considerably the frequency of premorbid diagnosis, treatment for tuberculosis is indicated in any patient with silicosis and a positive tuberculin test.

Other less hazardous silicates include Fuller's earth, kaolin, mica, diatomaceous earth, silica gel, soapstone, carbonate dusts, and cement dusts. The production of fibrosis in workers exposed to these agents is believed to be related to either the free silica content of these dusts or, for substances that contain no free silica, to the potentially large dust loads to which these workers may be exposed.

Other silicates, including talc dusts, may be contaminated with asbestos and/or free silica. Accidental exposure to significant quantities of talc may result in an acute syndrome with cough, cyanosis, and laboured breathing (acute talcosis). Severe progressive fibrosis with respiratory failure may ensue within a few years. Far more common is the fibrosis and/or pleural or lung cancer associated with chronic exposure in rubber workers who use commercial talc as a lubricant in tire moulds. Pure talc does not produce fibrosis; thus it is difficult to sort out whether the effects are due to the contamination of commercial talc by asbestos or by free silica.

In nature silica is closely related to calcium. In our time calcium is the main constituent of the animal skeleton. In a former period in earth history Calcarea silicata was an important element. Here silica starts to become a part of organic life instead of inorganic compounds. One of the most important parts of organic silica we still find in the sea environment. The biggest part of silica is coming from the rivers and when arriving in the sea is taken in by the animals to build up their skeleton. Then there is a deposit of silica on the bottom of the oceans and the rivers too. And another part is coming to the surface and used by other animals. So when you consider the first rudimental structure of animals skeletons, e.g. of sponge, the prominent part of this skeleton is a kind of spine, the structure of silica is a kind of spine in the skeleton of the sponge. There is a classification of the sponges. While the very basic sponge contains a lot of silica, the more developed sponges contain less silica and more calcarea. So in nature the change from silica to calcarea is a step forward in evolution. It shows that silica was much more prominent in the old plants like equisetum, which is a very ancient plant. In the times of dinosaurs there were much more plants containing silica. So it is a very basic and ancient element.

Discussion of Silica themes

STIFFNESS/RIGIDITY

Rubr.: **obstinate**
Inner resistance and stubbornness, inflexible, rigid, stubborn and fixed to certain images, which Silica wants to fulfil. Fixed ideas and just two possibilities - yes or no, it is this or that and nothing else. For Silica it is very important to fulfil this fixed image, to live like this. He also does not want anybody else to leave this way.

Nails and teeth

The organs of defence - <u>nails and teeth</u> that come under the influence of this remedy – are used to maintain himself in this stubborn way. Silica is very inflexible, cannot assimilate his system, he cannot bend, just break. He is like glass. Only when melted it is flexible, in this stage you could perceive it as yielding but when it is cold, it just breaks. It is so important what others think about him. He is not creative, not producing, but rigid, black and white, reproducing in a very perfect way.

Defensiveness/ nolimetangere

Rubr.: **Mind anger, contradiction from contradiction, intolerant of**
Violent when cross. When someone attacks her in her opinion, she feels like acting violently. But she cannot express her irascibility. She feels her weakness so overwhelming that she cannot show it. She is especially vulnerable to injustice, but she can express this only in a socially accepted way – not like Causticum, but more like the Kalis who have the idea of what is right and what is wrong and are not able to act different then according to this idea.

Rubr.: **Desire to kill**

Violence is not one of the main themes of Silica. The acting out of violence is forbidden, it is suppressed. For this reason the irritation of Silica is easily to distinguish from the irritation of Tarantula, Belladonna, Nux vomica and Hepar sulfuris. Silica reacts much slower. For them every injury is not only a physical problem. As their structure is so thin, so untouchable, so inelastic, it is not easy to cope with it. They lack elasticity so much, that an injury could break the system.

Rubr.: **Mind, contradiction, intolerance**
For every remedy in this rubric this intolerance is in accordance to different kinds of the self-perception. E.g. - *Aurum* feels the contradiction directed against his plans . For Silica this contradiction threatens directly their structure. In Silica the injury goes much deeper. I have to defend myself, I need to be a kind of porcupine. It is not possible to endure any kind of injury. So this idea of yes and no is very prominent. As we saw before, this acting out of violence is forbidden and we consider a very slow system. So, when you quickly hit them their specific reaction is to become very hard. The theme of the needles often is coming up.

Rubr.: **Fear of needles**
This rubric could be a symbolic summary of their perception. They try to resist to any kind of injury, and a needle is even more difficult to control because it is so subtle and could easily penetrate your system. A punch you can expect as an injury, but to see a needle in time you have to increase your capability of looking around you. When even a very small stuff like a needle can injure you in a very deep way you can develop a fear, like an elephant could have in front of a mouse.

We have seen this being so stubborn, resistant and rigid, and on the other hand we find this soft side.

Weak structure

Lack of self-confidence, combined with weakness. There is a strong fear to fail, to do something wrong described in the Rubr.:
mildness
yielding disposition
holding, being held ameliorates - expression of the need of support

magnetised, des to be
anxiety about trifles
conscientious about trifles
remorse about trifles
fear of failure
timidity, appearing in public
ailments of anticipation

Unreliable support

He needs support in the sense of a fixed structure and not so much in a healthy relationship. He is so anxious to fail, to do something wrong, that his structure could be in some way injured, each decision could be a possible failure, everything could in some way destroy his structure. This structure is so fixed, so untouchable, it can be damaged by the slightest injury. Even a contradiction is a serious threaten.

desire to be magnetised
anxiety about himself
anxiety in chest during menses
anxiety from noises, from disturbed sleep etc.
contradiction intolerant

PRECISION

fastidious, obstinate
conscientious about trifles

The way of being stubborn in little things: it has to be like this and this. Once again this black and white perception in common daily things, e.g. children putting their cars exactly in a certain line or corresponding to the pattern of the carpet. Putting it in a certain structure. For them it is a great problem that what others consider a trifle is not a trifle at all. What a creative person can adjust, Silica cannot. There are a lot of anxieties and little delusions and a feeling that is a kind of being persecuted. Every little thing, something like a needle, for Silica is a fundamental danger to his structure. He is so weak, mostly in his mind, so he has to take care for every single piece of his puzzle. It is the idea that when you take off even one brick, the house is damaged and can fall down. It is not like this in Nux vomica or Aurum or others. So the matter is that what for other people is a trifle, for Silica is not at all. Also a small stupid matter could be a possible injury for the system. The idea is to save what I have, trying to take care of my poor energy. This attitude is also seen in the importance they give to the theme of money.

Restricted environment/ withdrawal/ hold in

Rubr.: **avarice**

del pursued, **fear robbers** is an important theme, the theme of money, fear of thieves coming to my house

delusions spectres, ghosts, spirits

Water:

dreams of a drowning man

Relationship to water is another important theme. Most of the plants, containing a lot of silica need to stay close to the water. Sand without water is a mass without structure. Together with water it can keep a certain shape.

In the process of Silica the relationship to water is expressed in problems with the kidneys. The relationship to water is also important to differentiate a silica process from other remedies

Slowness

mind: retarded children
dullness, sluggishness
slow dentition
slow respiration
fever adynamic
slow development
complaints of bones
injuries, bones, fractures, slow repair of broken bones

DD Calcarea carbonica – Silica:

All these general themes you can also find in Calcarea carbonica, but in which way is it expressed in Silica, which kind of difference we can find? A weak structure, desire for support, a kind of slowness, need for defence, need for a structure, chilliness, perspiration, and much more we find in both of them. Important is the way of expression of symptoms in the repertory. For working with themes you need a precise idea. You need to consider these themes in a specific context. It is not so easy to have this consideration.

Homoeopathically talking, which possibility do you have to make a differentiation between the many weak remedies with an apparently childish system? In which way can we consider e.g. the childishness in Silica as childish? Calcarea carbonica and Silica are both belonging to a very basic system. You can find them often together. Not only in Calcarea silicata but in many other remedies we have the same very basic structure, their dreams and delusions are just around that. So it is not a creative mind, not at all. Silica needs a very specific support, morality is yes or no, he does not need to understand something, he just wants to know what he has to do. They cannot use their mind in a creative way, but in a very analytical one. You have the example of their thinking when you consider a computer. They consider themselves a genius. At their small field of understanding they look very deeply. The matter is that I work with the data and the data is my mind. So, according to the few data I have I give the maximum and I give the best. The problem is that outside of this data I cannot cope with anything, this is too complicated. So this is how Silica thinks normally. They overwork, they overdo and they are really very good in their small field of existence. In their pattern they are always very good. They are very analytical, they can give you a precise idea of what they mean what is the reality of this problem. From this point of view they can be very premature in comparison with the Calcarea personality. The problem is that the point of view is very strict, narrow minded, because what is important is not to enlarge my possibility of understanding of my environment, but to go deeply into the few things that for me are really important. So they can get very fanatic persons, the fanaticism is close to the mind of Arsenicum. As silica is contained in the skeleton, it is an inner house, an inner vertical structure on which you can grow. It is a male structure, but in a very basic sense. The shell of Calcarea is a house that protects you. So Calcarea has this possibility of a home, but in Silica any support is lacking. For this reason they feel weak. Often this is a delusion, they are often very intelligent, but they feel weak in their body, cannot perform the basic male approach. That means he must be intelligent, means to become a premature man. One could say Silica wants to be nursed by the father. Silica has no home, always exposed, must always show who he is, he feels how stiff and easy to break he is, like a crystal. There is a complete lack of elasticity, they look strong because they are so simple. They are obstinate in going their own way, they are proud about their products, e.g their stool, whereas Calcarea is obstinate in his well-known forms where he feels save. Silica thinks he has to become perfect in his limited way. They try to show what they can. They want to give the impression of a structure that they create inside themselves. They restrict themselves to be very good in this small field. Then it looks as if Silica could be like Baryta carbonica. He is restricting himself because it is clear in his mind that he cannot do anything better. In Calcarea carbonica it is a fact that they are not intelligent enough, for Silica the problem is that they feel very weak. They show a very basic male attitude, feeling that their body, their muscles, their physical possibilities are not strong enough. They cannot cope with this natural weakness of a growing system, they try to compensate this lack of strength with intelligence and perfection in their specific field.

Relationship with food: we find a strong aggravation from milk in Calcarea, a person getting allergic to milk. A person who wants to be breastfed even if is he is not hungry. Calcarea cannot endure to be alone, needs somebody who takes care of him, a fat baby that needs mothers breast. They acquire their milk allergy after having had too much of it. Calcarea is a person who wants to be a child forever whereas Silica wants to become a male as early as possible. For Silica a social idea is unimportant, a tree can only remain in one place. The structure is vertical, in Calcarea horizontal. Both need practical support and money.

Image / split

Silica has a lot of **splitting tendencies** in the mind as on physical levels. They are the expression of inflexibility in combining two things, only yes or no is possible. They know very clearly that they show to their surroundings a different person as they are at home where they choose a weaker partner because it would be too stressful to keep up their image all the time. In the very few dreams and delusion that they can report this fear to be discovered and injured is evident. Even a small thing as a needle can be dangerous, not easy to be seen, so one must always be very alert.

delusions: being on two places in the same time, being double , divided into two parts
left part does not belong to the right
sees robbers in house, will receive injury, about pins, someone is behind him
dreams: robbers, fighting with, having been betrayed, neglected business, being murdered, pursued

Hold in

The idea that you have to be conservative, that you have to preserve, is one of the main matters. They must over control the situation. In my understanding together with the Kalis Silica and Silica-like remedies represent the most con-servative persons you can find. I am not talking about the political point of view. It could be something like this too, but the idea is that they do not want to change their lives and themselves, it is too risky. The main quality of them is to preserve.

Vexation

Rubr.: **Anxiety of consciousness** - is another term of a theme of persecution
"Feelings of guilt" belongs to the fact that you have to do it properly in a very rigid way, when moving away from this very rigid pattern, there is persecution. Sense of guilt less in the sense that you did something wrong and someone else has pain or sorrow. This feeling of guilt seems to be only about themselves, without sympathy. It is directed towards an over asking father who will punish him if he does not do what he asks in a proper way. In this sense they can also be religious people.
A bit different is the feeling of *Bambusa*, who wants to be recognised for what they are doing .
Kalium bromatum also has to fulfil the desire of his awful father. In the case of the Kalis it is a much more elaborated problem, they are less stiff and less black-and-white than Silica. In the case of the Kalis the feeling of guilt has its

origin in something deviating from common thinking in society. The Kalis are very aware of what is going on around them in their conservative circle of society. For them law and tradition at home and in society is very important and they want to remain attached to this kind of ideas. Anything new could be a serious problem.

Restricted environment

Rubr.: **Selfishness**
In the case of Silica you do not have this problem about society. The main stuff of Silica is that it is self-referring. They do not care so much what is going on around them, what is going on in society. They create their own narrow, fragile, strongly severe, strict environment and they need to remain attached to that. They are overreacting to anything that is not in their direction. They don't care so much if this model makes sense or if other people accept it - not at all. This is an important DD from other remedies.
Both, a Kali and a Silica person could become fanatic, but they would probably choose different religions: The Kali person could develop fanatic ideas in the common religion of his region, the Silica person would choose an individual path. It is not so easy for Silica to cope with and to compare himself to other people while in the case of the Kalis you need to meet with the rules, you need to be recognised as a member of a society. In the case of Silica you are a single element, a person on your own.

Summary of Silica themes

Weak structure
STIFFNESS/ RIGIDITY
Image/ Split
Restricted environment/ withdrawal/ hold in
Unreliable support

Defensive, nolimetangere, poor defence
Slowness
Chilly
Bones/ nails/ skin/ connective tissue
PRECISION

Insecurity

Vexation/ dreams of vexation

Enlarged head/ rationality

Water/ weeping/ perspiration/ urinary tract

Allergies/ milk (unreliable support)

BAMBUSA ARUNDACEA

Description of the substance

There are about 50 genera and more than 1200 species of bamboo. The exact botanical classification is difficult, taking its cue from the blossom's structure. Various kinds of bamboo blossom rarely - some only in intervals of 120 years. Bamboo is an evergreen plant, though in some species some of the leaves become yellow in fall, remaining on the branches together with the green leaves. Bamboo is very resistant. After Hiroshima's destruction by the American atom bomb bamboo shoots were among the first plants emerging from the soil. The bamboo plant comprises underground rhizome, calm and branches. The calm, stem consists of joints and nodes from which the branches will grow. At a very rapid rate of growth (20 - 50 cm a day!) the joints open like a car aerial being extended. While growing, the joints are surrounded by a cane sheath containing growth hormones. Later these sheaths are dropped. (Bernd Schuster). The young shoots have already reached their full width (up to 20 cm) when they emerge from the ground. They won't grow any thicker. The number of segments between the joints (internodes) is already fixed within the shoot. No later growth in height or width is possible. However, higher and thicker new culms are developed each year and also the number of branches increases. There are no branch shoots until the cane has reached its full height. (Bambusa arundinacea grows to about 8 metres.) Bamboo wood is made up of 1 cm long fibres, whereas wood possesses fibres of only 1 mm length. These long cellulose fibres are packed with lignin and silicate dioxide, or silicic acid. The culm, having reached a certain height, starts to bend slightly. The usually longish leaves sit on a stem. Inflorescence comes as broad panicles. Bamboo's fruit almost always appears as berry shaped caryopsis (dehiscent fruit).

The flowering intervals range between 1 and 50 to 120 years. Some species are in blossom synchronously in different parts of the earth, whether it is they stem from the same clone, or due to other still unknown reasons. Flowering is a great strain for the plant and usually – without fertilisation – is either followed by slow growth for several years, or an increased rate of death, because all reserves stored in the rhizome have been exhausted. The bamboo plant is very hungry and very thirsty. It needs lots of fertiliser and a lot of water, as the leaves evaporate a colossal amount of moisture .

Bamboo usually multiplies by growing further rhizomes, or by separation. Some species have invasively spreading rhizomes. Untended groves can double its root area every year. This vigorously spreading variety is called "running" bamboo. Underground barriers are used to keep them from spreading. A few hardy kinds of bamboo and most tropical species grow in a much more re-strained fashion. The rhizomes of these non-invasive, "clumping " kinds of bamboo grow only several inches (1 inch = 2, 54 cm) a year. (www.halcyon.com/abs/BarnhartIntro.html)

Chemical analysis of Bambusa arundinacea (according to Wehmer): Cane con-tains pentoses, hexoses, N-compounds including choline, betain, CHN-splitting glycoside. Shoots: nuclease, urease-like enzymes, (...) salicin slitting, laevo-rotary reduced sugar.

Edible bamboo shoots

They are not lignified shoots of the genus Phyllostachys, especially Phyllo-stachys pubescens, etc. They should not be eaten uncooked, as they contain a poisonous cyanide glycoside, which is destroyed by heat. (also contained: ben-zoic acids).

The proving substance Bambusa e summitatibus (of Bernd Schuster's proving) is produced from the fresh growing tips of Bambusa arundinacea, triturated for three hours. One should consider that B. Schuster's Bamboo-proving was done with a quite poisonous substance.

Tabashir:

The name Tabashir (or Tabaschir) derives from the Sanskrit word "Twak-kshira", roughly meaning bark milk. Tabashir (also known as "vansa rochana") is a crystalline substance, which is found in the lower internodes of various species, but never in reed - like bamboo. 1830 Geiger reported: a sweet juice oozing out of young stems at the nodes is collected as bamboo sugar (Tabashir) when hardened. It is extremely precious and is valued as highly as gold. The root shoots are preserved and eaten, a luxurious confection (Achier), as gastric tonic. According to Tschirch's handbook, there are two types of Tabashir. The first can be found on the stem's surface (...) the second inside the stem. The first kind contains mainly cane sugar, the second silicic acid. (Schneider). Tabashir contains up to 92 % silicic acid and is obtained by burning the cane.

The burned concretions are dirty grey and converted into a "milky white, opaque or bluish-opalescent chalcedony-like mass(...)by calcinations (Warburg).

Tabashir: (...) 1% water, 99% SiO_2, plus traces of iron, calcium, aluminium and alkalis." (Simonis).

Traditional use

Parts of the bamboo plant are used in folk medicine for the following indications:

Leaves: blood diseases, leucoderma, haemostasis, promoting menstruation and lochia, vomiting blood, vermicide.

Branches (decoction of the tips) and swellings of stem: uterine complaints, abortive agent, inflamed joints

Shoots: respiratory diseases, to aid digestion, wound cleansing, gastric tonic. However, the non-medical use of shoots as vegetable is most typical.

Nodes: uterine activity, promoting lochia, regulating scanty or irregular periods, abortive agent, and ointment for inflamed joints.

Root: against ringworm, a ring-shaped fungal infection of the skin and other skin rashes

Flower juice: diseases of the ear and deafness.

Bark and seeds: snake bites.

<u>Tabashir</u>: blood diseases, tuberculosis, asthma, leprosy, cough, gallbladder dis-
eases, antipyretic, aphrodisiac, paralysis, consumption or emaciation, flatulence,
chronic dysentery, internal bleeding, epilepsy.

Technical use

In Asian countries bamboo is used as building material; water pipe for irrigating
fields; raw material for paper; for household matters like ladders, receptacles for
food and drink; for music instruments (pan-pipes), for manufacturing high-
tensile ropes and as food. The cane even is used as scaffold for high buildings.
The leaves make excellent "seed free" mulch for annual gardens.
Bamboo can produce 10 times more cellulose material per hectare per year than
even fast growing trees like Pinus radiata, doesn't require any heavy machinery
to harvest and is easy in usage and handling. Other ways to make use of bamboo as living plants include nutrient uptake in wastewater, erosion control,
windbreaks, hedges and many, many other kinds of usage. In Columbia bamboo
is used for replanting riverbanks due to its dense rootstock holding the soil in its
place. This is why bamboo groves are said to be the safest place to stay during
an earthquake. There are also earthquake-proof bridges and houses made from
bamboo.

Myths, legends, ritual use

Bamboo is supposed to bring luck throughout the whole life, if the umbilical
cord of the newborn baby is severed with a bamboo knife.

In ancient China people identified with bamboo, which was seen as the very
symbol of the Chinese character. Bamboo stands for suppleness, endurance and
perseverance. Its stems bend in the wind but do not break. The leaves are moved
by the wind but do not fall. Bamboo yields and this is exactly why it survives –
becoming the victor. In Japan this characteristic is still referred to as "bamboo
mentality": reaching compromise, giving in, but ultimately emerging from all
troubles unbroken. The bamboo cane is as strong as steel but more flexible.
When exposed to heat and then bent, it retains its shape without loosing its good
properties such as suppleness. In China bamboo is a symbol of modesty, because its heart is empty, of old age, because of its evergreen leaves, and of
laughter -bamboo doubles up with laughter, as B. Schuster reports.

In Japan it is a symbol of family. Out of a network of roots grow different generations of stems; old plants and shoots are coherent through their roots.

Toxicology/ Pharmacology/ Medicine

Experimental medical studies have proved the following effects: action against tumours, sarcoma 180, anti-inflammatory and anti-ulcerative effect in gastric ulcers, reduction of gastric acid secretion, antitussive effect, effects on leprosy. It contains an estrogenic active constituent and causes infertility in male rats.

In Morbus Bechterew we find the x- ray terminus of a bamboo like spine (German: Bambusstab) because of the analogy in the appearance of the ossified spine to a bamboo stick.

The proving

In 1994 Bernd Schuster conducted a methodical large scale proving of Bambusa arundinacea. The potencies - C6 Q3 C30 dilution - were made from fresh bamboo shoots. The proving was done with great precision, every word literally recorded, summarised and statistically evaluated. More than 50% of the persons taking part in the proving dropped out. The proving symptoms were observed over a period of 2 months.

Main themes coming up in the proving:

Mind
dissatisfied about the way life is organised, desire for change in life
feeling overworked, overloaded, exhausted, and stressed out, also by their own child.
despair, need of support
irritability, quarrelsome, wants to be alone, to be quiet
feeling things are getting on top, not able to figure things out
need to get rid of excessive baggage
difficulty finding the right word
depression, laziness, sadness, weeping at night
fears: cancer, aids, vertigo, something wrong in the head, etc.
forgets names and words
difficult to concentrate, cannot find the right name

fears being observed for the condition, losing self-control

And on the other hand:
capability of decision taking increased, more independent
more self-confident - perception of inner feeling increased, feeling of inner harmony
increased energy, vigorous
less influenced by negative daily events
less fear and more relaxed
dreams of water, of waves, of the Arch Noah

Vertigo
as if coming out of the neck
wavelike movements arising from legs to spine
when bending, sensation, legs are moving and bouncing up and down
fear of vertigo
Head
dullness, empty feeling, sensation something moving inside to the right eye
"balloon filled with hot air"
Headache
tearing to the **eyes**, extending from the neck to the front
pressing, during stiffness in the neck and back with pain in the extremities
menstrual headache
Vision blurred, foggy diplopia at night
Nose discharge, coryza obstruction, sneezing
Throat
inner: swelling for days, raw, sore, feeling of mucous
external: swelling of thyroid, cannot bear anything around neck
Stomach.
nausea comes in waves
heartburn after wine, beer, sweets, excitements, fat, beer, meat
desires cheese, wine, cold water, and fresh stuff
thirsty for warm and cold drinks
increased appetite

Diarrhoea
strong urge, frequent defecation during the day

foul smelling flatulence

Female
menses painful, dysmenorrhoea, menses during lactation
painful swelling of mamma
menses appears stronger

Back pain during menses
decreased or increased **sexual** drive

Back
"Stiff as a stick"
pain in the cervical region, unable to turn the head, warm bath amelioration
stiffness, extending to arms and hands, shoulders, scapula
stiffness lumbar, sacroiliac junction, better warm application
problems with inter articular discs, bamboo – spine
distinct tendency to support the head

Extremity pain
wavelike pain

Shoulder joints, often with stiffness of joints of knees, hands and feet, back lumbar and sacroiliac junction

Pain is mainly stitching, sharp and short, suddenly coming and going, sciatic pains.

Discussion of Bambusa themes

Weak structure, unreliable support

They feel they are not capable of carrying too much of a burden, too many duties or functions; they feel overloaded easily; have brought too many things down on their head. They can bend for some time, but then it is too much. In Morbus Bechterew we see a spine that is fixed in its bent position, where they cannot get up anymore. There is this feeling of too much weight sitting on their neck, producing many neck symptoms. Many fears related to the possibility of decompensating and loosing their image, if others see their weak spot or their sickness - for example fright or perspiration.

Fear of loosing self-control, fear of a break down, cannot handle things any-more, conscientious about trifles, lack of self-confidence. So they despair, be-cause there is no possibility to get help from outside. It is very difficult for them to accept help, because they burden themselves with every possible weight. They do not find any support because they cannot ask for it; there is a big fear of loosing self-control and that others might observe their weak condition. As the plant in its compensated state, the patients carry and bow and lift up again. They can grow over their own measure, like bamboo that stays flexible as long as it has enough water.

Water

They need a lot of water; as long as they have it they can bend. We find a clear relation with water, also with waves. The theme can be expressed in the rubrics delusions, dreams and vertigo: dreams, **waves moving through the head**. Even though bamboo is such a strong plant it is of utmost importance that it has a lot of water and rich soil.

The numerous vertigo symptoms could correspond with this uncertain ground and the fact that bamboo plants are flat rooted, despite the height of their stems. Bamboo has a very a characteristic resistance to a special kind of situation, but the plant itself is very sensitive. So it is not that simple to just say it is a strong plant. When they are worn out, they loose their flexibility: the head of the bam-boo hangs down, as the patients very often will support their heavy head with their hands during the consultation. But even then they rather would not change their inner concept. Their Silica - like rigidity shows itself in this point. Their inner program and plan of growth and development cannot be changed by any-thing, so they stubbornly stick to their way, which they have started to develop from a very early time on.

REPRODUCTION/ FAMILY

For these people it is not easy to connect with their surrounding other than their own family who lives in the same ground and comes out of the same "rhizome". They are strongly connected to the soil, often living in the same place all their life and feeling homesick when on vacation.

For bamboo, reproduction takes a lot of energy, which we can also find in this remedy. The bamboo grows up and blossoms only very rarely, maybe after a hundred years and after this period it is completely exhausted. On the one hand they might keep up their program blossoming at the same time all over the world; on the other hand it is very difficult for the plants to flower, and when it happens it takes so much energy that the plant may die. Family and children take a lot of energy and the patients feel them as a big weight on their shoulders. Their fears are directed towards their children and whether they will be able to take care of them properly. So the family theme is very prominent.

DD Bambusa - Silica: In comparison to silica it is striking that bamboo is a plant and does not show a crystal structure. Rather it has an organic part that makes it more flexible and more communicative, as Silica has no relation towards its environment. Bambusa can at least communicate with those who belong to her family and to her closer surrounding. A special relation to her surrounding is expressed in the rubric: **the wedding has to be repeated; only half of the body has been married** – which also gives a hint to the tendency to split up. This is common with Silica. On the physical level they share coldness and sweating.

Bambusa has half its symptoms in common with Silica. Just making a numerical relationship, it is interesting that a plant like bamboo has so many symptoms in common with the crystal silica.

VEXATION

In M. Mangialavori's cases fear of vexation and anger is a very important theme. Anger was not expressed and reported very well. Often the information came from the patient's partner rather, than from the patient directly, who would talk about other topics. But it seemed to be evident that there was a person with a deep problem not easily expressed.

MODESTY

In some cases it was really impressing that the person was too calm when reporting about a serious pathology. One would have expected much stronger complaint, e.g. in a disk protrusion this person could only move like a Bryonia case because of serious pain, but reported the situation very calmly. He tried to go on in his habitual behaviour - as if the body was something separate. He wanted to appear absolutely harmless, like a monk, like a person who does not care about himself. These people always agree, talking very shy with a low voice. They really need to show they are modest. Through their mild, calm, soft attitude it is not so easy to see their other side, which they only show towards their husbands/ wives or other close persons.

Numbness

Numbness is an important theme, but unlike remedies like *Laurocerasus* or *Opium*, where a lack of perception of pain is common. Here we find an evident discrepancy, a split between talking and a strong physical reaction. M. Mangialavori reported that his patients where like that in their common life too. It was amazing how a person with such a vexation - a situation where many other people react in a very severe way, were apparently not able to react.

VICTIM

On the other hand pathologies, ailments or severe physical conflicts are found, that make the patients unable to express themselves. They try to remain the same or to pretend that nothing is wrong and they never want to present themselves as a victim. But normally they have the tendency of becoming a victim of other people or of a situation in some way, and they feel like a victim but would never admit it. "I am strong like a bamboo in the storm, it does not matter." Quite often you find Bambusa patients living in awful situations. *Bambusa* has more tendency to relate to his or her surrounding, which makes Bambusa a victim, while *Silica* is much more reluctant to enter a relationship with others; they rather withdraw as much as possible from every environment, that could be dangerous for them.

M. Mangialavori's Bambusa cases are very good in their profession; again they are less narrow-minded than Silica. In their own field of work they are really among the best, it is important to them not to be like the others and they want to be seen. They can have ambition as can be found in other remedies like *Natrum*, *Aurum* and *Nux vomica*. But you will never find a Bambusa boss, a person who is able to perform and to appear in front of other people. They always complain that though they do such an awful lot, though they work so hard, they are not appreciated enough and that other people take profit of their incredible capacity. Both remedies - Silica and Bambusa - lack the capacity to be able to firmly take hold of a situation, to say: here I am. They want to appear masculine, like a person who is able to act, to produce, but they do not succeed in being recognised. They are not successful in a sense of **Veratrum** or **Aurum**. Bambusa patients are flexible, can adapt to any situation, but finally they are unable to express who they really are. Bambusa hides weakness by bending too much; Silica does not show weakness by being rigid.

Image/ Rigidity/INABILITY TO MOVE

With their strategy to compensate their weakness both of them become absolutely strong. When you dry Bamboo, it is like steel and provides a very strong material, hard and useful. The stronger the mineral side, the less flexible it becomes, the less the point of view can be changed, the less thoughts about their environment can be modified. Due to lack of self-confidence they need this overprotective structure. **"That's how I am and I won't change"**, is a keynote of Silica as well as Bambusa and all Silica-like remedies.

M. Mangialavori's cases of Bambusa were real workaholics. They really showed how professional they were, but were always victims of someone taking profit of them. There is not one single case of Bambusa who worked alone. Like cases of **Ambra grisea** or Silica they worked together with a stronger personality who was often a member of the family, but with this tendency of taking profit of them. Their only reaction was to increase their professionalism, their capability to understand what was going on. So they often became real specialists in their work field, trying to do their best and complaining about nobody appreciating this fact. It is very rare to hear this directly from the patient; usually the information comes through very close friends, or the doctor's clear perception. Or there must be a very close relationship, or something like a confession.

They are so stoic, you could think that it has to do with their dignity. But their dignity is pretended in a sense, that it really is the person's self-destructive way of showing she or he is strong enough to endure the situation. They give the appearance of a modest person, who couldn't care less, able to endure everything, while on the other hand, they really suffer without being able to express themselves.

34

Unlike Silica, Bambusa is not so narrow-minded. But from a certain point of view both are very stubborn and fixed to their ideas. It is not so easy for them to change their pattern of becoming victimised. As within the plant, the complete information lies inside the rhizome. According to its inner rhythm it will start growing like an unreeling program. In bamboo the quantity of internodes is fixed from the beginning, the diameter of the young pipe is the same as of the old.

Again, when you have a discussion with a Silica patient, usually they react strongly or leave the discussion. Bambusa people are always like a Chinese person, giving you a nice smile and saying ok, you are right. And then continuing in the same direction like before, following their inner pattern and never changing their mind. Both cannot really cope with other people, but Bambusa hides weakness by inner inflexibility, bending as much as possible and pretending to be strong, whereas in Silica we can directly observe its stiffness and rigidity, as Silica is always aware of his/her weakness. Silica expresses narrowness and stiffness while Bambusa´s self-image is: I am so wide, so supple.

In most of the Bambusa cases suffering was a physical representation of their inability to change, to move from a certain situation. They remained in the same place in the common Silica way. Often they developed symptoms obliging them not to move. Inability to move is a characteristic pathology. To move away from a certain situation to them means giving up a certain position. This is one of the very common organic representations. Any motion, any movement increases the pain. With any back pain one needs to remain absolutely still; so often they want to remain in a very hard bed or – seen with 3 Bambusa cases - they lay on a table, suffering in a very modest way, showing: this is my habit rather, not really masochistic. They choose something very hard, need to stay in a very hard situation, and they feel that not moving is the adequate reaction in such a hard situation. The desire to remain in bed during illness is also very evident. Averse to being disturbed, they want to do whatever they please in their own way. So also their obvious fear of a crowd is understandable. The stiffness of Bambusa is a spastic reaction trying to hold back or to hide something, mainly represented in the back muscles. They suffer from alternating neck- and lumbar pain.

Motion agg.

Pain is perceived as paralysing and they must lie down without a single move-ment. They suffer deeply. **Bryonia** has the same tendency of keeping everything inside with no desire to move, also the same tendency with money, the same kind of avarice. But with Bryonia you have more arthritic pain and inflamma-tion, as well as infectious diseases. With Bambusa you find a more mechanical, degenerative problem. They pretend that the pain is not affecting them much, but of course the stiffness is a never-ending story: the stiffer you become, the more pain you have. It becomes a common habit and so they develop a severe pathology, but try to show that they are not so sick.

Chilliness

Normally there feel very chilly and coldness worsens the pain. But if they catch cold and develop diarrhoea, they often feel better.

Discharge amel

Often they feel an acute amelioration with any kind of discharge, mostly when they can evacuate or have a diarrhoea pain ameliorates. - reported by 3 patients. **Equisetum** has the same amelioration with discharges, but more represented in the urinary tract.

Slow reaction

Bambusa is very stoic and doesn't like to change a situation.
Characteristic of Bambusa as well as of Silica is the problem of suppuration, of infection. If we consider a slow reaction a must for the Silica family, we cannot restrict our observation to slow healing suppurations, which we know so well from Silica. First of all, today we do not see this kind of suppuration anymore because it would be treated with antibiotics. The slow reaction should be seen in any other process, as it should be a clear mind symptom. Because of the pre-tended flexibility we don't have the same kind of slow reaction with Bambusa as with Silica. Because of its hardness, Silica is not able to repair done injury. To injure Bambusa is much more difficult, as she will apparently change her attitude and come back to her starting point

For example, with male, respiration, cough, extremities and skin you find lots of Silica symptoms, while in the throat and, not only by chance, in the back Bambusa is predominant.

Summary Bambusa themes:

Weak structure
Stiffness/ Rigidity/ INABILITY TO MOVE
Unreliable support
VEXATION/ SUPPRESSED ANGER
MODESTY/ VICTIM
Slow reaction

Water
REPRODUCTION/ FAMILY
Chilliness

Pain cramping/ paralysing/ numbness
Neck, spine
Degenerative processes
Discharge amel, esp. stool
Motion agg

M. Mangialavori's first Bambusa case

M. Mangialavori reports: It was not easy to get any information because the patient was a very reserved person. He is one of the mildest persons I ever met, behaving like a monk really, always smiling very nice and sweet; and I never heard him quarrel or rightfully ask for anything, though he worked in an environment where a quarrel is very common. He is an electronic and network specialist, very renowned and very good. What's interesting, on the other hand, is that he works together with his brother, who is very different, only 2 years older and much less professional. He is not able to work with the same precision, but has all his brother's sympathy. And he really takes the profit of him. For years now they have been working together. His brother has a nice villa, a beautiful car and became rich, while my friend still drives his awful, old car. He doesn't have a house so it's evident for everybody that one person is taking nine parts of the profit and the other one. Nevertheless he has never been able to react. Often all his friends told him, how good he was, that he could work less and earn more money, and asked why he was doing this. He said he didn't want to have discussions concerning his family, his brother or his parents; he didn't want to show them that his brother was like that. When I met the patient he had been divorced for a very short time and again his wife took all the money they had. She didn't work and took all the profit of him. When I met him he was acquainted with another lady I knew quite well, because she was a patient of mine too. They stayed together for something like a year and practically never had sexual intercourse, because she had problems with vaginism and for her it was impossible to have sexual intercourse. All the time the lady thought she had to see a gynaecologist, and every time she had a haemorrhage she kept fainting. I could treat her successfully with Bellis spinata. After three years with this lady I treated him. The problem was that six to seven times a year he had to remain in bed completely paralysed. He couldn't move at all, had two burgeons, one in LWS5/S1 and the other in the lower LWS region. So sometimes very easily with a single movement he remained completely blocked and every time he had this, he lay on the floor or on a table, not showing any pain even when it happened. Later he got married with another lady that was well treated with Pulsatilla and in this family not even a single bad word was spoken. They just talk and laugh, absolutely not Italian, they are like two Japanese. I treated him for years using common remedies for his kind of vexation, and I struggled a lot, because none of the remedies I used worked. I sent him to an osteopath were he was treated very well. So he felt better, but still he came again.

As soon as he was able to move, he got back to work, even if he had to work only for one or two hours on his computer in the office. His secretary was always very rash with him and completely on his brother's side. So, that's what the situations was like. One day I was completely desperate, because they called me again I was just studying bamboo and I thought, what an interesting remedy. I considered everything. But I never had described the remedy before. Anyway - I gave it to him.

Luciano, aged 38

His hair is completely white. He is of small build, talks in a very precise way, and is extremely shy and mild-mannered, giving the impression of a humble, weak person. Very precise answers .He looks prematurely aged, older than 38, more than ten years, walking, moving etc. Tries to excuse his family even considering his bad situation

*** 'I was diagnosed with several disks' hernia, and I have had many different treatments.

It began when I was only eighteen. I've always had a very stiff back, and ever since I was little they told me, mine was like the back of an older person. I've tried various treatments, but I'm not an athletic person. The only thing I like is sailing, but I could never do it regularly because I feel the cold too much.

??- It regularly locks up and stays locked up for days.

??- The only thing I can do is lie down on a hard surface. First I used to lie down on the floor but it was very painful when I had to move and get up… then I thought of something rather unusual but more practical: the kitchen table. I live on my own and so I can do it. It's only a problem when my parents drop in to see me, or one time our secretary came by to tell me what phone calls I had to make. Well, of course they thought it was rather strange. You don't usually use the kitchen table to sleep on…

I have to lie on a hard surface, even though my head and back feel like solid block… ??- I can get locked up for the most stupid reasons. They told me to be careful, that I wasn't even a candidate for surgery… however I wouldn't let myself be operated on even though it's crossed my mind more than once because now it's really got to a point… if I couldn't do my work any more it would be a disaster… it's the only thing I know how to do and I stuck all of the little money I own into my business.

??- The first thing I notice is a freezing cold feeling inside and if I can make it in time I quickly go and run myself a nice hot bath… if I manage to I can avoid locking up completely. ??- My whole back hurts but my neck is always stiff as a board and I can't even move my head… then the pain goes downwards and starts hurting me lower down and it goes all the way into my arms and hands. And then it goes to my lumbar area and I can only walk with a hump in my back because I can no longer hold myself up straight. ??- It all contracts and I can't move. Sometimes it becomes one solid mass… and I can't bend over any more, because if I do I can't get back up…'

??- ** 'Apart from this I've had a headache for as long as I can remember. I've tried everything against that too and at the headache centre they say it's mainly caused by muscular tension. But that's what they say now. Before, they said it was a kind of sinusitis and before that it was something else, I can't remember what they said…

The first time they took me to the doctor's for a headache was when I was six years old. I remember it well because it was my first day at school. I've had it ever since. I would get an awful lot of mucus and even my ears would get blocked up and my stomach got upset and a whole load of mucus came out of my nose… but only after days of using aerosol inhalers and baths and going to hot places and to the sea. Fortunately my parents have a house in Liguria/ Italy and we often went to the seaside. I would lie in the sun on the beach and my brother went off to play with his friends…

He often underlines the image of his brother

??- It's very painful, and my neck feels as if it could fold up like the handle of an umbrella… ??- I mean that it doesn't bend, but I have to hold my head with my neck bent forward so as not to feel the pain so much.

??- I can't take any kind of chill, not even in summer – especially not then. In winter it's normal to be well wrapped up. The pain goes up from here, my neck, into the whole of my head, which feels like bursting.

??- Apart from the cold the other things that make it worse are… always before I take an exam… always, that's guaranteed, and I get diarrhoea too… and also whenever I've finished doing something important…

??- I love my work, but doing what I have to do takes a superhuman effort.

??- I can't do anything badly: *I'm very precise*, and I'm also told that I'm even stubborn. I work in information technology, I began with *writing programmes and then installing systems*. I work with my brother, he takes care of running the business while I look after the clients… It's hard work, but I like it a lot.

??- EVERY time, I mean EVERY time that I do a new installation it has to work perfectly, and it does, but then I get a headache. The more demanding my work is, the worse my headache gets… It's like a barometer of how much effort I have to put into everything.'

He has to swallow holding in a bad feeling and it is like pouring gasoline into a fire (Italian expression)

??- *** 'I get satisfaction from the work with my clients. ??- I get on well with my brother, but it's hard to get on with all this competition and I'm not such a pushy person…

??- Unfinished business with people bothers me. I used to wake up at night thinking of something… I'd carry on ruminating on it and feeling bad about *it…seems that I cannot say I'm giving more gasoline into the fire than there is inside myself* it's a matter of learning. I'm the calmer type, whereas my brother's quite adventurous…'

*** 'I also had something very strange: a small induration, which they said, was a sort of fibroma on the mammary gland, and I also had gynecomastia when I was a child. Now it's the size of a small pea, I think about it even if I don't notice it. It got a lot bigger three years ago when I learnt that my father had intestinal cancer.

??- I realise that I could easily have it, but I have these pangs… But he had lost the will to live…'

*** 'Recently I've been very worried about my family and also about some of my friends, even some of the clients I get on best with. I see some of them every week… I think a lot about how to mention it and the fact that their health could be at risk. ??- I would like them to tell me. ??- Not in a rude way… I don't like it at all if someone is rude to me. ??- It just makes me despair.

I remember I went to a healer… he didn't talk that well, only in dialect, and he told me I had a lack of energy. I do so many things and don't get tired easily… but then I get a headache or my back locks up…'

What is seriously disturbing at the moment?

??- *** 'I've started to think about death almost obsessively, more so as my parents have grown old… lately I've been thinking more about it. I think I lack the ability to evolve a certain kind of spirituality. Thinking about this subject makes me feel egoistic and that I'm doing it only out of my own needs. I HAVE TO BRING FORTH THAT WHICH IS CONSUMING ME, I have to but…'

his concept: feeling to have the need to trust someone, no real trust in god. Than changes topic again

*** 'I tend to get constipated and I often have to help myself to pass stool. I often have to help myself manually to get it out.

??- For a long time…??- I've had the urge to go in the morning and when I was at school I used to hold it in because I couldn't go to the toilet and for such a long time I think that was bad for me. I held everything in, and in the afternoon it's difficult to go.

Now I go to the bathroom in the morning, but often its difficult to go… perhaps it's because I'm impatient… but I have to go to work and I never have time for these things…'

Problems when younger?

??- ** 'It was getting a problem that I wasn't growing a lot and I had been physically very precocious… my genitals were already developed at the age of ten. My precocious physical development blocked me emotionally… and I held everything in. I was taken to an endocrinologist and I didn't eat very much, I only ate chocolate and they made me have a GH growths hormones (somato-tropin)…something that's antagonistic to gonadotrope hormones)

??- I don't think it was a good thing for me because then my headaches got much worse and I will never forget that they ruined my back.'

??- *** I also had asthma: what was worrying was that it was impossible to breathe normally. Then I discovered I was allergic to grass pollen. Now every spring I get crusts in my nostrils… always in spring, or if the temperature changes and it lasts for months. My voice gets very nasal and it's tiring to have to go to work like that.

??- My nostrils get small darkish crusts in them, and above all my mucus is dry… when I had sinusitis I used to fill handkerchiefs with a foul-smelling yellow smelling catarrh.

??- I pick them off and they bleed a bit.

??- Chocolate has always been my passion and I think I must be addicted to it.
??- Obviously plain chocolate, the kind for connoisseurs… Otherwise food is optional, doesn't matter to me.

It was an incredible reaction, not only because in a short time he had no pain any more, but for the first time he was better and after three days in bed, he decided to have a vacation with his wife instead of coming back to work as he used to. In the following time they decided to have a second child; while before his wife virtually had to pray to him to have one. And this idea of not having a child had been one of the main problems causing the divorce of his first wife. She had wanted to have children, but he said he didn't have enough energy, not enough money, he didn't feel secure enough. Now they did not only decide to have a second child, but in a very short time, he had a reaction very well known for **Staphisagria**, an incident with his brother, when, in a very cold way he practically destroyed his office. They had a discussion and he just - not like Nux vomica or Hepar sulphuris.- took calmly the computer, opened the window and threw it out. They separated with the help of a lawyer.

Follow up
After taking Bambusa Q1 for 4 weeks he had another backache. Stopping the remedy, he had no backache for 4 months (they often react to treatment after a long time (slow reaction). Then relapse after a quarrel with his brother.
Therapy: Q1 every hour

Control in the middle of spring: I had no allergy, no headache.

I had the feeling of being the little baby of a bear. I am very fond of bears, but to me they are unreachable. I love how they hibernate and are able to endure cold; they even can swim under the ice. The Panda is my favourite animal and I am very fond of bamboo. I like to eat in Chinese restaurants. I felt less chilly, without sinusitis and flu. I worked very hard without pain and it was as if something was missing (no pains). So I have my bed on the table no more. My back is much better, I feel more flexible; before I was hopeless, I can move much better. Before I felt I had to open a knot, something in my spine.

??- I feel a strong responsibility for my brother, I am the youngest, and I have a good sense of reality. My brother even can quarrel with a saint, so we loose a lot of good clients. Financially we were bankrupt twice only because of him. Even the bank account is done by him and the secretary, who is his lover.

Vexation of him was clear. He cannot handle it.

He drives a Porsche and I a Fiat Uno. I don't want to think about what this means to me.

The real goal would be having my own company but I cannot stand being all by myself, although I could have less stress and my spine would be much more supportive.

Therapy: higher potency.

Two months later urgent telephone call because of a severe state:

I called my brother, he said: "I am sorry, but I will go to the seaside with our secretary".... and at this moment I couldn't move anymore. So please help me.
Last night I dreamt I couldn't walk. I had to reach the hill of Golgotha, so I wanted a stick as support, but there was nothing, only a small plastic stick they sell for kids, it was not strong. Every time it touched the soil it made a noise like making fun out of me. I kept walking like an old man and each time I heard this mocking noise, so I thought it would be less humiliating to crawl, which I did... Waking up I felt stupid.

He is not at all recognised by his family. Whereas his brother even could have been put to jail. So it actually felt less painful to him to endure his situation, rather than to endure what happened afterwards.

After the Q3 he went directly to the lawyer and broke his relationship with his whole family.

From then on up to now he has hardly suffered of any backache, he only had three relapses so far and every time Bambusa is working very well for him. The osteopath had asked, "What did you give him?" because before he had hardly been able to work with this man, and now the muscles were smoother and the situation a lot better.

Second case

This woman was a well-known specialist in her profession. She came to be treated because of a big fibroadenoma in her left breast and she was in panic about it.

Several times she would have had the possibility to become chief of her department, but she refused to. She even could have worked as a free lance due to her high professional qualities, but she never had wanted to. She didn't even remain with her boss, but kept changing from one chief to the other, but the situation got worse every time.

She decided to get married only at the age of thirty-seven. She said, until that moment she hadn't felt mature enough. And the main problem had been, that all the men she had met wanted to live a very strong, adventurous life, whereas she was a very calm person. The only men she had met before had been too stressful, doing a lot of sports, and also the last one, the person she decided to marry, was a person with a lot of influence, as she was too. He went parachuting, sport skiing in the mountains, climbing and indulged in quite a few other kinds of sport. What made this relationship really important to her was, that for the first time in her life, she said, there was a person who was able to listen to her.

"I am a person who has never been able to express what I have inside and this is like putting gasoline on a fire that could destroy me. For the first time in my life I have been able to choose a person who will listen to me. Try to imagine I wanted to check if it is possible. When I wake up from my sleep and something is crossing my mind I can wake him up and we talk about it."

So she reports this as being amongst the matters of utmost importance when choosing this person to live with. The main reason for coming, she claimed, was because she was in panic due to a fibroadenoma in her left breast, that now had become very big and had appeared when she got to know of her father's abdominal cancer. She said the only therapy that had done something for her until now had been acupuncture, having made her a lot better and reducing the mass of the fibroadenoma but the problem was her panic, because her mother had had cancer and had been operated on and two of her mother's sisters had had cancer. She had always had a severe swelling in her breast before her menses, which had always been a serious problem for her, but recently it had been really painful. Mostly since she had had this all the time, she said she could continue to live with it, but it was kind of a menace, gnawing at her.

??-How do you react when you have this feeling?

"The first reaction I feel is a severe stiffness, because every time the idea crosses my mind my reaction is to block my spine. If I'm lucky I only have a severe pain in my cervical region and I prefer to have it because it means I only can't move my head. I become very chilly. I can't move at all. I have to lie down on a very hard surface; often I put my blanket on the only table I have, in the kitchen, so they have to cook in the same room and they have to eat in another room because I can't move from the table. The first severe reaction I had was in my adolescence; but the first time I was really obliged not to move for two weeks was, when I got Hepatitis B and they forced me not to see my daughter for a few weeks to prevent an infection and it happened during the first period of my marriage."

When she suffered this she felt such a strong pain that she had to remain like that for a couple of weeks.

So asking some questions about her relationship with her daughter, she said:
"I came back to work when my daughter was only four months old. My parents transmitted this idea to me so after that moment of stress I got the Hepatitis. I think the only way for me to allow myself to remain at home was - to be sick. But I was punished, they took away my daughter. A severe problem for me was that during that time she was much closer to my mother and in the end she called for my mother instead of me. And she never wanted to come to me tell me anything.....anyway for me it was a disaster.

"My parents are getting old and what I feel is very bad, that they miss a certain kind of spirituality and I feel I am a very egoistic person because I am not able to make them aware of how important it is to have a spiritual life.

I think having a spiritual approach to life gives you a feeling of immortality. Nobody can touch and nobody can change it. You are always the same forever, but the problem is, when this kind of secret is not affecting you, but is affecting friends of yours or parents it's really bad, because they are not able to change."

Another common problem is, that she suffers of obstruction in the nose since she has been a child:
"It is really severe stuff for me, because I have always the need of expressing what's digging at me, breathing as I like is something awful, because I have the feeling I cannot take it."

When M. Mangialavory wanted to have more information about this the patient was not able to express herself. At a time some years ago, when she was pregnant, she had been treated by another homeopath and he had given her a different kind of Kalis (bichromicum, carbonicum, nitricum), because she had this problem of obstruction, with a lot of pus and very difficult to detach, she took this remedy also for her backache and nothing changed. It had always been a problem to go to the toilet, she always had to take some purgatives, and sometimes she even had to help with her hands:

"It started when I went to school because for me it was impossible to go to the toilet in school. So I was obliged not to go and slowly, slowly it became a habit. The problem is I always have the desire to have my stool, when I cannot follow it. For example: in a situation where I cannot find a toilet, and if I can find it I am not able to make it, I must be at home. One of the most important problems of my life ", she said, "is, that I was not able to grow, even though I was very precocious, because at the age of ten I already had big breasts and this was a problem for me because I used to do a lot of sports. I used to behave like a male and to keep everything to myself and I really suffered a lot. Everybody made fun of me, because I was so small and it was decided to treat me with a growth hormone."

I forgot to tell you that she is only 105 cm tall.

Another problem she has now is that she has to urinate involuntarily, and to her this is severe, happening most often when she sneezes, and she tries to sneeze to relieve her problem of the nose obstruction. This involuntary urination is a symptom of Bambusa too and obstruction of the nose is a symptom of Bambusa, mainly when you lie down. I did not take all the symptoms of the fastidiousness and of the stiffness of the back and the symptoms I already knew of Bambusa, because I was thinking of it.

Until now she is very well with this remedy. Her situation changed in such a way that, for the first time she decided to take the courage to start her own business, which was kind of a milliard stone, for her family too. First it was a problem because her husband complained that she was more out than at home. The anxiety about her fibroadenoma then had become much better; it was not cancer. At another time it was shrinking and remained smaller for two years. The problem of urinating, the obstruction of her nose and her constipation ameliorated strongly. Her sensitivity to cold still remains; when she doesn't wear a cap it is common for her to start sneezing, but then she takes Bambusa, which helps her in a short time.

Impressions of these two cases:

Delicate patients, peaceful, quite ambitious, but not standing up for themselves; they don't show how much they suffer. She refused becoming a boss because it wasn't the kind of work she liked. She wanted to work being a doctor and not a boss. "I prefer other people, having a more precise attitude to do this work", she said. It is evident that she was unable to express any kind of healthy aggression. She blocked her back at the same time as she was separated from her daughter. Bambusa has a close relationship to the family.

Ailments from anger and vexation:
The first back pain happened when she felt the danger of being separated from her family. The rest of her family, mother, father and some cousins never supported her to become a professional in her specific field. This was one of the main reasons why, even if she had decided to do something different, she was practically obliged by her family not to do this because they were very frightened that she could not fulfil everything.
It is very easy for others to take profit of them. This kind of people seems open to help you in every possible way, even if you don't ask them. When they think you would like help they will do whatever you want, but they won't change their attitude.

Additions of M. Mangialavori for Bambusa

- BACK; PAIN; General; Lumbar region, lumbago; cold, from taking
- BACK; PAIN; General; Lumbar region, lumbago; sneezing
- BACK; STIFFNESS; Cervical region; headache, during
- BACK; TENSION; Cervical region; headache, with
- FACE; ERUPTIONS; acne
- FACE; ERUPTIONS; acne; forehead
- Face; ERUPTIONS; pimples; forehead; painful
- Face; ERUPTIONS; pimples; painful
- Generalities; FOOD and drinks; cheese; desires
- Generalities; FOOD and drinks; cheese; desires
- Generalities; FOOD and drinks; meat; aversion
- GENERALITIES; FOOD and drinks; sweets; desires

- GENERALITIES; WORN OUT
- MIND; FEAR; panic attacks, overpowering
- MIND; RESPONSIBILITY
- MOUTH; APHTHAE
- VERTIGO; MOTION; from; vomiting and nausea

EQUISETUM HIEMALE

Description of the plant

Plants of the genus equisetum are also called SCOURING RUSH, 30 species of rush like, conspicuously jointed, perennial herbs. Equisetum is the only living genus of the order equisetales and the class sphenopsida. Horsetails grow in moist, rich soils in all parts of the world except Australia. Some species produce two kinds of shoots: those with cone like clusters (strobili) of spore capsules and those lacking such structures. Some are evergreen, others send up new shoots annually from underground rootstocks. Their hollow, jointed, ridged stems contain silicate and other minerals. The leaves are reduced to sheaths that clasp and encircle the shoots. A widespread species along stream banks and in meadows in North America and Eurasia is the common horsetail - equisetum arvense, about 30 centimetres tall. The central cavity of each stem is about a quarter of its outside diameter. Fairly thick, solid branches arise from below the sheaths, circling the shoots like spokes on a wheel. Stems that bear terminal spore cones are often flesh-coloured. Wood horsetail - equisetum sylvaticum grows in moist, cool woods and has many delicate branches that circle the shoots. Variegated horsetail - equisetum variegatum is evergreen and has black markings on the sheaths. Dutch rushes - equisetum hiemale, common in moist woods and on riverbanks, reach well over a metre in height. The evergreen shoots often are used for scouring. Giant horsetail. - equisetum praealtum of North America and Asia, which reaches 3 1/2 metres (11 1/2 feet), also is ever-green. Each shoot has as many as 48 ridges. The giant horsetail of Europe - equisetum telmateia is about the same height as Dutch rush. The tallest of all horsetails is a slender South American species - equisetum giganteum, which sometimes grows to 10 m (about 32 ft) in height with a diameter of about two centimetres (less than an inch) and is supported by the tall grasses or shrubs around it.

Equisetum hiemale and equisetum arvense are the only used species and therefore described further on: The light type is growing on the meadow and the bigger ones, the dark green ones are growing in the wood. The plant has a big rootstock, a rhizome, out of which grow the shoots in spring. They do not contain chlorophyll. This spring shoot is only there for 5 or 6 weeks to build the sporangia and the spores. Then it dies and out of the spring shoot there comes a summer shoot, which is very similar to the spring shoot in case of equisetum hiemale while the summer shoot of equisetum arvense looks like a bush. Equisetum hiemale calls to mind the bamboo. It has no side branches like the Equisetum arvense. We do not know why the homeopaths chose this species; nobody in the herbal medicine ever used the equisetum hiemale. It was only used for cleaning tin dishes; therefore its German name is Zinnkraut. It has the highest content of silica and to cut the herb is difficult, whereas on touch it feels astonishing soft.

There are several names for the plant: Pferdeschwanz, Katzenschwanz, also Schachtelhalm, because its end can be extracted out of the sheets of leaves between the internodes and can be replaced again. You can manipulate it from the outside, but also easily break it. In its aspect it has some similarity to the bamboo, but the stem of bamboo does not break so easily, it is elastic.

Equisetum is considered a weed, not useful, and it is an indicator for wet soil. Even on a dry surface it indicates water. The relationship to water is one main theme going through the remedy picture. Relationship to urinary tract, bladder, kidneys. As bamboo they need a lot of water and a rich mineral soil, so its growth is a sign for water and for rich soil, from which they use up many minerals.

Equisetum is a very old plant, so it has not a developed system. In the past this plant was enormous, what we are using now are just the children of equisetum. Sometimes you can still find the big ones. In Bolivia M. Mangialavori found an equisetum giganteum, eight meters high. In this case one could see the similarity to the bamboo, even if it is a different plant. Like bamboo is an evergreen. This idea of being evergreen with this continuous need of lots of water is a matter that belongs to very old plants and is characteristic for those that do not flower. The more evolved plants have a different relationship to their surroundings. They are more adaptable to nature and they change more. Gymnospores and conifers are the most ancient plants. Like Lycopodium they are an old and inflexible system. The faster plants grow the more they have a flexible relationship to their surroundings.

Contents and toxicology

The older the plant gets the higher is the content of silica. Equisetum hiemale has even more silicic acid then the others. It has a crystallised form, which is the same like in Opal.

We find saponines, several organic acids, calcarea, potassium, sodium, manganum, magnesium salts. The alkaloid equiesetim is sometimes considered to be the reason for intolerance in cattle and also people, and this is a different explanation than in Reference work where equisetum is considered an antidote to herbal fungus in gardening and in alternative farming because it is resistant to any fungus disease itself. Ustilago is a very frequent contamination of equisetum. It is said that equisetum is the bread of the horses and the death of the cows. This means is a good food and hay for horses but has often bad effects on cows, they loose their teeth and get other sorts of complaints. Only special sorts of equisetum like equisetum palustre etc cause the toxic effects on cattle and man. It is not clear if equisetum itself is poisonous or only getting poisonous when contaminated with ustilago.

Traditional use

Some species are utilised in polishing tools because of their abrasive stems.

Information about the plant and the use in herbal medicine can be found mainly in Europe. The plant is known since ancient time. Though it is considered a small remedy it is reported in many books. The Latin name equisetum hiemale means horse's hair in winter. Horsetails, although poisonous to livestock, are used by man in folk medicines. The herb that is used in herbal medicine comes from equisetum ardense, and only homeopathic medicine uses the species equisetum hiemale. Herba equiseti where made out of the equisetum arvense and used for lithemic conditions. It was used for gallstones, concrements, joint problems, but mainly for the treatment of disturbances in the urogenital system, and it was considered a diuretic.

The old Romans said even holding the equisetum would stop the bleeding of a wound immediately.

The German parson Kneipp used it extensly for his blood cleaning therapy, but also for many other indications as tuberculosis, skin disorders, coughs and all kind of lung problems because of the high content of silica.

The American Indians also used it for burns.

Some of the effects can be understood from the contents of the plant: malleic-, aconite-, arsenic acidum. The acid explains the strong stimulating aspect.
From the content of iron, copper, calcium it is easily to understand why it was useful for anaemic people. Used for all kinds of bleeding, very astringent.

Rudolph Steiner gave it some reputation for being an alternative remedy against fungus. The founder of Anthroposophy - held series of eight seminars for progressive farmers in 1924. He wanted to explain his ideas in their own language and his lectures were put down by hand, later transformed and printed. Steiner had the idea, that man, plants and animals, as well as the inorganic world were related to and dependant from each other, and the whole cosmos with moon, stars and planets too. Concerning equisetum avense he said when there is a very wet spring and wet winter, and there is much water in the soil, the energy of the moon influences the soil too much. So all seeds get stuck on a lower level of the plant and they cannot develop properly. They are on a second level offering soil for other organisms like parasites and will be eaten by them. To prevent this you have to protect the plant from the moon energy and that is what equisetum can do. So the decoction of equisetum came to alternative agriculture. When you see the first louse or parasite in the garden you put equisetum in your rainwater and then you water your plant.

There is an interesting use of the powder, made from the trituration of the dry plant, which can be used to stimulate the growth of hair and of nails. Horses were fed with very small quantities of the powder when their ankles were weak, or when they had problems of easy ruptures of tendons and of weak hoofs. With an ointment, made of pigs fat with powder of equisetum they used to brush the horses.
The powder is also given as a source of minerals to men, especially in the convalescence of tuberculosis.

From the alchemical point of view the dry part of a plant used as a powder increases the mineral side and stimulates the convalescent energy. In contrast, to use a lotion or put the dry plant into water changes the effect. The liquid part of the plant can treat stones of the bladder, kidney etc. A proving of the trituration would probably show much more symptoms than we know already from the tincture.

Case 43a, female, physiotherapist

She appears as very weak, fragile, face pale, thin face, as if fat was missing, not really emaciated but really lean, talking in a rough way sharp expression, very direct, almost giving order, sitting distant from desk in a kind of suspicious appearance, communicates with a defensive attitude, frowning.

"I decided to come for a consultation because of my gynaecological problems. When I had my last ecograph they diagnosed a uterine fibromastosis. The gynaecologist told me I have an age-related condition and that there was urine retention in the bladder. However I hadn't gone to the bathroom first, and I was sure my bladder was not empty, but he didn't want to listen to me. DOCTORS NEVER LISTEN TO YOU.

My mother had a hysterectomy because she had heavy bleedings. I only had one haemorrhage, after I gave birth. There was more than one liter of urine in my bladder and then I had to catheterise myself for two weeks because I couldn't control it any more. When I was growing up I had to urinate frequently. Although I had tests and urographs they never found any particular reason for it. I went to the doctors very frequently when I was little because I often had to go to the bathroom and the teacher used to make fun of me about it. I had used to wet the bed up until I started menstruating I even get it sometimes now if I have strange dreams and now I also have uterine fibromastosis. My periods started when I was 13. They were always very heavy, and my cycle was less than 20 days. Ovulation was always painful. I had a cyst 6 cm large on my left ovary. I always had a headache at the time of my period. My temple would begin to throb near my right eye and then it would go to my forehead. It was almost always connected to my period – either before or during it. If it's bearable I just hang on: I don't like medicines and doctors.

It gets worse from the stress of travelling or if I eat between meals: I'M A VERY PRECISE PERSON AND ANY CHANGE IN MY SCHEDULE CAN BRING

ON A HEADACHE OR SOME OTHER PROBLEM. But if I am in my own environment then it doesn't lead to a worse crisis... I can't go out of the house, first of all because the slightest draft of air makes it an awful bt worse. I have to cover my forehead... and then the pain goes to the nape of my neck and down into my shoulders, which turn into two pieces of frozen, lifeless marble. I cover up and wait; sooner or later it passes everything passes. The worst thing is this feeling as if I was in a boat during a submarine earthquake.'

Well, I was told that you have to tell the homeopath everything I had a difficult childhood: my father used to beat my mother or he came home drunk. We children grew up in an atmosphere that wasn't very tranquil. My mother was unhappy with her life; we were together just because we were a family. As soon as we could, we children left home. I have no relationship with my parents or my siblings. There were several suicides in my family. What affected me most was my uncle. He slit his wrists, and then he spent more than thirty years in a lunatic asylum. Then he came home and he got on well with me, I often used to take him out for a walk. When I got married he tried to return to the lunatic asylum but they wouldn't have him back. I HAD A FEAR OF GOING MAD WHEN I WAS LITTLE; I ALWAYS USED TO TELL MY MOTHER ABOUT IT.

When I was little I always had problems with my throat. They operated on my tonsils twice and then on my adenoids, but now I always have swollen lymph nodes under my jaws. Every spring I get bronchitis and then cystitis. As a rule I finally always give in and take antibiotics. I don't know if I got worse because of the bronchitis or the cystitis, but I am always very weak in those parts. I had cystitis when I was in hospital giving birth, but I blamed having to use the bedpan. I had another bout after my first sexual relations, and every time I had sex for more than a year after my wedding. The pregnancy was a very difficult time from that point of view... the vomiting apart. As I told you, I always had urinary problems...(*seems very embarrassed about I*) I always have to urinate very frequently... I'm not very good at holding it, and I wet the bed for years. Even now I can't retain it very well... and as soon as I get the urge I have to run to the bathroom, even if it's only to pass a few drops.... [*she is very embarrassed*].

I had many problems at school because I was often absent due to illness and this had a serious effect on my self-confidence. When I had my first son I had alopecia and then I also had it afterwards when he wouldn't take the breast. I had it at other times too. I took it very badly and it was lucky that the dermatologist held my hand and said it was just a psychological problem. Then my hair grew back I NEED REGULARITY IN MY RHYTHMS… if I eat a sandwich in hurry or when I'm coming home in the afternoon I always get a stomachache. I have cramps, with the feeling as if my stomach is swelling I feel wind going into my intestines, and I would like my stomach to be pressed. I feel like a very insecure woman. I don't feel steady on my feet, and I think it's due to how I feel inside. I have had so many tests for that. It's true that I am weak, but I don't think it's just that, I have gone on so many courses in which, when we looked into it, they showed me that my postural problems were only due to how I see myself It's difficult to explain. I was born old, an adult. I never had a childhood, and when I had to give birth, I felt as if I had already given too much, and I didn't have anything more to give to anyone… I don't have any energy of my own and I can't have any for anyone else… I find it hard enough to look after myself. I have to look after myself, life taught me that…

I do this work to help those who can't stand on their own two feet [*cries*]. You don't know for how long it was a real nightmare for me… I even dreamt at night that I was falling… I couldn't stand on my feet because my legs felt like bread-sticks… or sometimes like tubes of toothpaste or cream… and if I wanted to make myself look nicer and use those beauty products then my legs got weaker and weaker. They saw me walking like that and I couldn't manage it and noone could help me… I woke up in the morning and felt exhausted… and my legs were really hurting me. I don't have much self-esteem… managing to do this work has been quite a feat. I really sweated bucket loads… it was very exhausting.

I have always sweated a lot, and in summer I have to drink lots of mineral water because my blood pressure goes down. In winter I'm very scared of the cold. My hands and feet are always icy cold. I know I was born a weakling… my mother always used to tell me that I was the most frail of all my siblings and that they kept me alive just because she wanted it. But it's very difficult with the way I am… 'I'm a very precise person… I'm very disorganised inside, and if I don't keep everything in perfect order, then I can't find anything. At work they tell me I'm a maniac… but the results are there to see… it's the others who see them though… I can never be satisfied with myself…I just can't do it.'

Main themes:

Weakness, inability to stand on own feet, so there is a need for structure, which is expressed by precision and control, urination problems, where normal control functions do not work, lifelessness expressed by icy coldness. Relations: not so submissive as people with a lack of security, but quite tough, so supportive to the uncle but she almost got crazy, when he did not want to go back...

Most problems on genital urinary tract.

Rubrics to be taken into consideration:

Weakness, enervation. {180> 478> 0} (Allen T.F.)

Weakness, enervation: forenoon: ten am. {0> 9> 0}

Weakness, enervation: waking: on. {5> 60> 0}

Delusions, imaginations: falling: he is. {0> 31> 0} (Roberts)

URGING TO URINATE, MORBID DESIRE: FORENOON: TEN AM. {0> 1> 1}

Urging to urinate, morbid desire: afternoon. {2> 11> 0}

Urging to urinate, morbid desire: night. {41> 70> 0}

Urging to urinate, morbid desire: constant. {0> 13> 111}

Urging to urinate, morbid desire: frequent. {28> 88> 100}

Urging to urinate, morbid desire: frequent: afternoon. {0> 2> 0}

URGING TO URINATE, MORBID DESIRE: FREQUENT: DESIRE INCREASES AS THE QUANTITY OF URINE DIMINISHES. {0> 1> 0}

Urging to urinate, morbid desire: sudden. {32> 42> 0} (Boericke O.)

Urging to urinate, morbid desire: sudden: hasten to urinate; must, or urine will escape. {26> 36> 0} (Boericke O.)

Urging to urinate, morbid desire: urination, after. {2> 18> 50}

Urging to urinate, morbid desire: women, in. {3> 15> 0} (Clarke)

Urination: dribbling by drops. {44> 81> 0}

Urination: dribbling by drops: senile. {0> 6> 0} (Phatak)

Urination: dysuria. {76> 88> 0}

Urination: dysuria: delivery, after. {0> 2> 0} (Clarke)

URINATION: DYSURIA: PAINFUL: URINATION, AFTER, AGG. {0> 1> 2}

Urination: dysuria: pregnancy, during. {0> 5> 0} (Clarke)

Urination: dysuria: strain, must. {9> 8> 0} (Boericke O.)

URINATION: DYSURIA: URINE, WITH PROFUSE. {0> 1> 0} (Phatak)

Urination: frequent. {105> 108> 0}

Urination: frequent: night. {19> 51> 78}

Urination: involuntary. {18> 71> 94}

Urination: involuntary: daytime. {5> 5> 0} (Boericke O.)

Urination: involuntary: night, incontinence in bed. {0> 22> 114}

Urination: involuntary: night, incontinence in bed: dreaming of urination, while. {3> 5> 0} (Boericke O.)

URINATION: INVOLUNTARY: NIGHT, INCONTINENCE IN BED: TANGIBLE CAUSE EXCEPT HABIT, WHEN THERE IS NO. {0> 1> 0}

Urination: involuntary: old people, in. {7> 18> 0} (Boericke O.)

URINATION: INVOLUNTARY: WOMEN, IN: INVOLUNTARY STOOL, AND. {0> 1> 0} (Boericke O.)

Urination: retarded, must wait for urine to start: pregnancy, in. {0> 2> 0} (Boericke O.)

Urination: retarded, must wait for urine to start: press, must: a long time before he can begin. {22> 25> 0} (Boericke O.)

Weakness. {5> 23> 46}

PAIN: GENERAL: CERVICAL REGION: EXTENDING: SHOULDERS: MOTION, ON. {0> 1> 0}

Weakness: knee: exercise. {0> 2

Frown, disposed to. {1> 13> 0} (Allen T.F.)

FROWN, DISPOSED TO: ANGRY. {0> 1> 0} (Allen T.F.)

Irritability. {139> 297> 0} (Allen T.F.)

Discussion of homeopathic symptoms and themes

In the repertory there is little to find. Half of the symptoms are the same as Silica. Many rubrics are in common with **Cantharis**, but besides this very superficial aspect it is very different. There is the tendency to hemorrhage and for dropsy symptoms. Important symptoms reported by Phatak are not only aggravation or amel from/with urination, not only feeling of burning, but general the feeling of weakness of this patient.

In the very few symptoms we can find in the mind, there are interesting themes in the dreams. In the cases especially in children M. Mangialavori heard about dreams of being threatened by too many persons around. Or crowds that were mainly composed by awful persons that could injure the patient or pursued him or could do something wrong. In general we find a situation like in Bambusa or Zincum where they have to show that they are able to do something but they cannot. Not always a real examination. I see this in several cases of Equisetum. The thought of loneliness, no connection. In my patients of Equisetum comparing it to Silica the problem of anticipation is much more evident in the sense of what can I do to face all this problems. Not that you have to show that you are capable, but just the matter to face a situation is the problem. This dream of being exhausted in my opinion is very important. They have a very active life in their dreams, normally it is a torment. I think Silica does not like to give attention to this part of life, I do not say Silica does not dream. They are more oriented to basic real themes, not to dreams or creativity or using the brain for something that is not clearly related to reality. Something I never understood is this rubric: sociability for Equisetum, I cannot say anything about the source of it. In Equisetum this

feeling of persecution

or that people could do something wrong to you, this feeling that you have to face society or a person that could over ask you is so strong that you can say this is their imagination, about this matter. There is more inhibition then in Silica. Silica fears the confrontation with other people. Equisetum is even preventing the reality of facing the situation.

In the cases of the children they had always strong parents, in the sense of dominating and over asking the child, especially the father, often in a very subtle way. I am not talking about a difficult personality like the parents of Solanacae patients, that are punishing him, it is more an intellectual kind of severity where apparently his father looks like a nice person, but they don't give enough attention to the child, they give him the feeling they love him in relation to his capability to be adult or to produce something or to seem better then he is. They do not give him the feeling that he can trust in himself, do not transmit him any feeling of security. His value is nothing when he is not able to do this and this. Very often they grow with this feeling of being insecure, thinking, that his father is a great person able to do a lot of things and they will never be able to reach this level. Possibly the father could be a weak person in society and is taking the advantage to show the other side to his child, keeping him always under control. The only possibility to show he is someone while outside he is weak. So this kind of inhibition is very important. They feel they do not deserve this support and normally they are not able to react to this kind of vexation in a sane way, as in Bambusa and Silica. But they are very precise in punishing their parents with their symptoms. Very common is this matter of enuresis that we see often in combination with constipation.

Enuresis

is a common symptom so strong as in some Umbelliferae like in **Conium** or in **Cicuta**. You can find this even in adult people. I have two cases of enuresis where I first gave Silica to one and Cicuta to the other. They had an obvious this childish aspect. They got married but never left their family, they just include the husband into the system, so this childish aspect can be important as in Cicuta. Silica and Cicuta did absolutely nothing, after Equisetum the enuresis was gone and there where some more changes. Before they even could not imagine having a child, it was too difficult, too much. They were two ladies at the age of 30 years with this problem of enuresis. My impression was that they used it as a kind of punishment, when they were not able to react according to their needs and feelings during the day, like a child I remember, where his parents where complaining that this enuresis was really something disgusting. They even tried to wake up their son several times at night So in all this families, in all Equisetum cases I have seen, it is as if they are doing this to provoke their parents with the specific intention of doing something bad, of offending the parents. In adults it is a symptom of weakness. It often happens in situations when they are not able to relate to a great stress. In these two ladies it happened every time they had a discussion at work, or with their husband, not just for one night, but also for weeks. Something that is not depending on my will. When they had this enuresis, in the morning they wake up with a feeling of having done something absolutely strong, which used up a lot of energy.

They are very shy to talk about their problem of enuresis. I remember one case of a homosexual man, 22y. He had an enuresis. We did not understand each other. He was telling me that it was a problem, he was ashamed for this, he was never able to confess this to his friend and it was a problem because he would have liked to sleep with him. He said I am so anxious, I have the fear it could happen.

M. Mangialavori thought all the consultation long it was a problem of pollution.

There is a very strong inhibition and during sleep they can release all this control and even during sleep they are acting against this great pressure, and then they feel exhausted.

Not refreshing sleep, aggravation after urination

They tell about very intense dreams which they cannot report precisely, they just say there is a lot of things happening, a lot of confusion, and they wake up in the morning with the feeling of a nightmare, they cannot relax in their dreams.

In the bladder region there are plenty of symptoms, one of the most interesting in my understanding is this distended feeling. It doesn't mean only that it is a good remedy for objective problems of not being able to urinate, it is deeper, a kind of

feeling of emptiness - distended feeling

Some patients do not have real problems of not being able to urinate, but the feeling that most of their body's energy was concentrated in that region and that they were not able to get rid of this fullness. As if there was a kind of constipation in the bladder, as if they were not able to express themselves properly. Often they complain about a strange feeling, about fullness on one side, on the other side when drinking so much or urinating so much they feel exhausted. They are complaining in the same way as *China* patients do, but not about stool and diarrhoea but about fluids. It is the contrary of what you can see in *Gelsemium*. They feel better urinating a lot. In Equisetum urinating is always a trouble. I would like to get rid of this tension, this fullness, but it is not so easy and if I urinate as normal it is not better. They have a problem to urinate and when they succeed, they urinate too much. It is a kind of contradiction: I am not able to express anything, and when I express something it is too much. I have to keep in my energy and if I keep in I feel constipated. Symptoms of pressure and close to this the feeling of fullness. Pressing pain, aggravated after urination. They are always in trouble about this matter around the bladder. Like an anal character but related to the bladder. Many of the symptoms are clinical symptoms but a lot are just sensation. Equisetum has the symptoms like a child of seven years, who complains that the flow of the urine is so low. I remember a child who felt ashamed because he was not able to piss as far as his elder friends.

Rubrics:

dysuria with profuse urine, involuntary urination
kidney, pain general; urging; urinate, to, during
kidney pain general; extending; testes, to
urethra, pain; general; urination; close of, at
The urine, more then having calculi, often was watery.
The symptoms are strongly affecting the masculine side.
Most of the pain is sore, bruised.

Pregnancy

On the female side a lot of symptoms are affecting pregnancy. Both Equisetum-patients never considered to get pregnant, for them getting a child was too much and asking them about this theme was like asking something very strange.
In **Silica** is more the problem of what can I do, I am not strong enough, it is a heavy burden. They feel a kind of anticipation because it is another serious re-sponsibility. They feel I am not strong enough, mostly physical, and obviously in a woman this is stronger because in the beginning a child is really dependant of her and this is a fearful situation for them. In the cases of Equisetum it was more then this, more related to the male side of a situation, to the idea that I cannot express myself, I am not able to produce another life. So it is not only a burden, it is something that is far from their imagination. To show your male side, to produce something in an active way, for Equisetum is much more a serious problem then for Silica, because in some way Silica is able with his fixed mind to find out his little space and to express himself. So you have the general picture of a Silica patient, but much more inhibited. For this reason I underlined before the idea, that a lot is expressed during the night with this kind of enuresis.

INHIBITION/FIXED SYMPTOMS

The child grows up with the feeling, you are demanding that I become like you and on the other side you tell me I will never be able to reach this aim. It could be seen as a kind of sadistic approach by a father who himself is a weak person in society, and his only way of taking revenge and to feel that he is a strong person is to keep his children always under control. Here he could be able to express that he is strong, while outside he is nothing. So what we find out, as a main concept in this child is this kind of inhibition in acting.

Weakness/spineless

As in the case of Silica and Bambusa, when you have this kind of tropism towards the kidney it is also common to have serious problems affecting the spine. Mostly you find this feeling of weakness – as I have seen in all of my cases – not only as a clinical symptom but also as a mental representation of this weakness. We have seen that in general there is a lack of being able to express who I am, my male power, and my capability of doing something. And often they are complaining that this feeling in their spine is as if it was an empty tube. It is something close to what we find in Silica and Bambusa, but less evident is this tendency of remaining stiff or being rigid to show how strong I am. You have a tendency of affecting the spine and the idea of heaviness and of a lump as we have seen for Silica and Bambusa. Motion aggravates, and they need to lie down, like Silica and Bambusa. As if there was a kind of weight on their spine, as if they have to avoid the effect of gravitation, so they need to lie down, always feeling there is a pressing weight. Lying down makes the situation much better. In the cases of Equisetum, close to Bryonia, there is this feeling that they do not want to move at all, often single little movements increase their pain.

Summary of Equisetum themes

Weakness/ spineless – spine as an empty tube
Unreliable support/ not deserved
INHIBITION/ FIXED SYMPTOMS
DICTATORIAL/ position, persecution

INCONTINENCE WITH CONSTIPATION
Emptiness – distended feeling
Water
Aching pains

Urinary tract

Pregnancy

Back

Unrefreshing sleep

Silica – Bambusa – Equisetum

In common is the anticipation in confronting other people, lack of self-confidence, chilliness, sensitiveness to cold, and the idea that you are not good enough, the idea that you have to be really fastidious in your little world of work. The general idea of weakness is related to the general feeling of wanting self-confidence, the idea of a system without minerals, without spine, without power. You have to be very cautious in giving out and expressing your energy like a car that is lacking gasoline. They are very careful what they are giving out to take care not to waste their energy.

What seems different in Equisetum is that it is more problematic for them even to express themselves in a very specialised field. They are intellectual people that do not realise anything in life. They develop many good ideas of what could be but are not able to translate this into practice. So this theme of inhibition arises.

For Silica it is not common to be so dictatorial, stiff and aggressive as Equisetum. Equisetum used to be such a big plant, and then it became so small as Lycopodium. An interesting signature: former huge plants often show a very defensive attitude. Mostly kids want to appear stronger, bigger, taller, a must for Equisetum!! They need an upper position to be not so easily attacked.

Silica would more think I am not strong enough, also physically. Equisetum really feels his inhibition. Many symptoms are affecting the back; important is their feeling of lameness. This is not only evident in clinical symptoms, but in general they lack the ability to express who they are. Their tendency of overdoing, of remaining stiff, of being rigid, of showing how strong they are is less evident than in Silica and Bambusa. As for Silica and Bambusa we find motion aggravates, and as Silica and Bambusa they need to lie down. Any kind of weight is to avoid. In M. Mangialavori's cases of Equisetum there is something close to Bryonia, with this feeling that they need immobility, not moving at all. Often single little movements are increasing the pain. Most often the pain is aching, the most important symptoms are aching ones.

Methodology:

M. Mangialavori gives a lot of importance to the description of the pain. In any remedy he tries to find out how patients describe their way of suffering. Try to understand what it means when something is stitching, burning, etc.! Normally the remedies with this predominance of aching symptoms do not give you a precise idea of a special way of suffering, but just the idea that it is too much. They cannot express it in a different way that they feel not to have enough energy. Aching symptoms mainly are in relationship with a general feeling of weakness. The most appropriate expression for Equisetum is that they feel spineless. Anticipation in confronting other people, does not describe the same kind of elastic stiffness as in Bambusa. Stiffness is not even expressed in Equisetum, it is the stage before. Silica on the other side seems much more direct. The feeling of inhibition is much more prominent in Equisetum. They are less able then Silica and Bambusa to show this weak side. Their kind of stubbornness is a very special one; they seem to be more stubborn in not being able to elaborate different kinds of symptoms. The tendency to remain for a long time in the same kind of illness is characteristic. The reaction of Equisetum is even more inhibited then in Silica. In some way Silica restricts himself to his own specific world where he tries to be very good. He has contacts mainly with one partner, mostly with a weaker one. For Equisetum patients it is even more difficult to find a good relationship. They are intellectual people that normally are not able to perform anything concrete in their life. They develop brave ideas how something could be, but are not able to translate them into practice. All Silicas are good professionals and e.g. in Equisetum they are very good in making projects, but what is lacking is the translation into something concrete. One patient e.g. was a technical designer for ceramics.

Equisetum can be considered as a kind of Silica, but much more inhibited. Most of their symptoms are not expressed. A weak person, complaining about his weakness, complaining that because of his weakness he is not able to do his duty, his daily work. Everything is too heavy, too much, even if they are very responsible. The sense of responsibility is something special. They are persons you can really trust a lot. But obviously for them it is always a tremendous work.

This symptom of enuresis is disappearing slowly while other symptoms may already have a clear amelioration, often symptoms on which they are not giving so much attention. They are really fixed upon this one symptom, as if it is not only pathology. The pathology is that they are fixed on their symptoms. I can say that this stubbornness is in some way the defence mechanism. To loose this symptom means for them to loose their capacity of relating to their surroundings. It is as if you cut the very few possibilities of expressing themselves, a certain way how they are. Normally what you consider a symptom, for them it is not always a symptom, it is a part of them; it belongs to their essence.

DD Equisetum - Bambusa

Bambusa has this expression of stiffness, this idea that they have to be strong, that they have to endure everything. They want to show in their stubborn way that they can stay in this system also when it is hard and painful. This is not part of the Equisetum pathology that from this point of view is closer to Silica. Even worse in the sense that he is retiring in an even smaller environment and lives more in projection of a fantasy world. So the somatic stiffness is not one of the most important points in Equisetum as it is so evident in Bambusa. They are much more stiff in maintaining their habits. They do not want to change because, like Silica they have such a small representation of life and of themselves. It was so difficult for them just to build this that when they perceive that in some way the therapy could bring on a change, it is a threaten to their very system. If I am so weak and it was such an effort just to build up this, what can I do, where can I go, where can I move if I have to change this?

DD Kali / Silica-group:

It is a difficult matter talking about the Kalis without being more precise. In the Kalis we have to consider strongly which other part of the remedy is related to potassium. But generally what I don´t see in Equisetum that I can see in all the Kalis is that they refer to the society, to a group of people. This is one of the main differential points to the Silica group who are self-referrent. The problem for the Kalis is their reference to others, so they have not only to stand up; they have to stand like the others do. They have to adjust themselves to a common sense of being to be sure to be the best. What is completely lacking in the Silica group is this ability to confront other people and to think that you could be like the others. When you are a Kali, you are able to share experiences with others. For the Kalis the social life is very important, to have a partner, to be mondaine and elegant, even if it is a stress. They have the theme of sharing with their friends, with people who support them. They need to be well considered in so-ciety, in their group, they feel they exist because of the others.

In the case of Silica or in the case of Equisetum the confrontation with other people is a serious problem. They are much more involved in their own very small and safe environment. So they are able to have this small life, doing something very small and precise and very well. You have the same sense of responsibility in Equisetum as in Silica. He could be a perfect secretary, but you cannot expect from Equisetum that he translates a thought into action whereas Silica can do it, but does it exactly in his way; he does not want you to change his attitude. There is only one way to make it, which cannot be discussed. You can ask them to do something but how they do it will always be their own way. Silica is very proud and will do it very well.

Equisetum is very good in making plans, is much more open to evaluate how it could be, is more creative in his mind. What is really missing is the capacity of action, of relating to something practical.

Differentialdiagnosis to **Alumina:** there would be a kind of glue with the mother, a viscid attitude, strong fusional state with the parents, while in a Silica-case there would rather be the aspect of an unreliable support. Unreliable sup-port meaning, there is not trust that would make the child grasp, it is more about having to trust his own feet, there is the same kind of weakness as in sea reme-dies but they have to trust themselves. They often get married with an even weaker person, this is a way to control the relationship; they can be sure, that this person will not overcome them and therefore the other person is not likely to leave them, because he or she needs them. It is a restricted environment, where they live: I know that I am weak, that I have to trust my own poor en-ergy; therefore I restrict my relationship with the world around me. Within the workplace they might be the best employees, the best technician though not in a very creative way. It is a kind of small, protected environment, where they spe-cialize and know the rules.

Silica-likes – relationship to parents and the doctor:

These people have no good relationship with their parents, and often they can-not establish a good relationship to their doctor as well. If patients never had the feeling of somebody really taking care for them, they reproduce the same situa-tion towards their doctor. They cannot trust you because of their sense of persecution and often cannot stay in the cure. This is true for Silica and Equisetum and many other remedies. In general there seem to be two possible ways of acting as a doctor. One could behave like a mother, the first person of care for the patient, allowing him to do everything he wants, like a mother with the attitude, I love you because you are there.

On the other side normally the father is the one giving you rules. For these Silica like cases this side should be more active in the doctor, to offer them, I can care for you, but you have to follow my treatment. There should be a kind of directive approach. You need to make the patient follow you. It was difficult for Silica to have a good relationship with his father, who was an over demanding authority who never let him do what he wanted, but still he always tried to imitate him and restricted his feelings as well as possible. He needs a strong person, but in the same moment he feels his weakness and inability to perform. So he is not able to trust in the doctor so much, he does not want to take remedies, doesn't like to follow your suggestions and you have to lead him very cautiously. You have to make sure to him that you like him and are interested in him; otherwise he will never be open to change anything in his life because of your directions. The idea of changing anything, leaving their habits, is the most difficult one for a Silica like person. The real beginning of a healing process in patients like this is when they are able to be a bit critical about what they did until now and when they can discuss about something that was a dogma before. They should understand that changing their habits could also mean changing to the better their pathology. For them this process is a very long one and therefore the Silica pathologies are always very long and slow.

In children I think it is the same. I have not the impression that this remedy e.g. in enuresis worked symptomatically. Because you know, there are so many children where enuresis is a severe problem. I consider that this is a kind of red spot, a good sign to think of Equisetum but not a very prominent symptom. This pathology is part of a dynamic process. Usually they have a long history of the problem, at least two years, mainly between six and ten years. Very often the parents tell you that everything was normal in the kindergarten and in school, nobody died etc., and Equisetum helped in this cases where you couldn't find any hint to a cause.

They are shy, have a lack of self-confidence. It is so difficult to enter into a relationship. Talking about a child we consider a patient who is not coming because he is feeling sick but is someone who is just brought. So you are starting from a very difficult point. Further they are often attached to their symptoms in a stubborn way, which is not easily changed. In some way for these poor people their pathology is a kind of structure. Especially here it is important to respect the symptoms. Taking away the symptoms is like taking away part of their person. With the progress of the treatment you see a kind of rebellion in Equisetum. The child is able to react in a different way. It can be similar after a treatment with **Natrum** or **Staphisagria** that the mother finds the child not so nice as it was before and you have to convince her that this is not an aggravation, but amelioration on the mind level of the patient.

The model of similarity

What is really missing in homeopathy is a well-organised model of thinking about what we consider a diagnosis and what is the relationship to the treatment. Diagnosis and treatment belong to the same process. If you have some results it is important to define why you have them. Sometimes we use one model and then another one, often very superficial ones like dividing human beings into categories of three miasms.

When you are studying a substance, as a starting point you have to define why Silica works and why not. It is necessary to come to an agreement about this in a group of some homeopaths. We try to find out a scientific explanation. I look at the way a certain system expresses itself. This is sufficient for me to find out something. But what is similarity; on which level can I consider similarity. On which basis do we define which are the main points of Silica, what is necessary to make a prescription of Silica. You find out very interesting remedies for differential diagnosis, as e.g. yesterday we talked about the differentiation between Calcarea carbonica and Silica. The basic symptoms could be the same and you have to see the context of the symptoms. You see why Silica is narrow and why Calcarea carbonica is not at all.

So I think important to have a definition of what we use for prescribing, because very often the definition of the remedy as we use it is only a list of symptoms. You can have 10.000 symptoms of Belladonna, but you need to understand what is really important to prescribe Belladonna and why and for what reason, otherwise with Sulphur and Calcarea carbonica you can cover enough symptoms, but it does not work.

So we think about the definition, what are the main topics for Silica. It is out of discussion that e.g. Lachesis and Silica are like two different continents, two different planets. We have to find out the minimum consense of a group, e.g. the most important characteristics of the Silica-like remedies.

SPHINGURUS MARTINI

Scientific classification:

Eurasian porcupines are referred to as the family of Hystricidae. American porcupines are referred to as the family of Erethizontidae. The common porcupine is classified as Hystrix cristata. Tree porcupines form the genus Coendou. The North American porcupine is classified as Erethizon dorsatum, the thin-spine porcupine as Sphingurus villosus, and the Amazonian porcupine as Echinoprocta rutescen. Mure described a kind of porcupine of that name, perfectly resembling Hystrix prehensilis, which inhabits Brazil and also uses its prehensile tail to move about

Preparation:

Trituration of the spines.

Description

Eurasian porcupines inhabit the forests of Southern Europe and Asia as well as those of Africa and Indonesia. American porcupines include four genera: the tree porcupines of Central and South America, the North American porcupine, the thin-spine porcupine of Brazil, and the Amazonian porcupine. The North American porcupine can be found from Alaska's wooded regions down to the Northern extreme of Mexico. One species lives on trees.

Characteristics of the animal:

Porcupines belong to the family of rodents, are some of the largest rodents and very corpulent animals. In phylogenetic terms they are very old, very slow animals - uncommon for rodents, who are normally quick and shy and don't dangle from trees or live in cavities. Porcupines are plant-eating animals. During the day they stay on trees and usually leave for their meals only. They eat fruits,

leaves, berries of all kinds, plants and also all materials made of wood, prefera-
bly salted wood – and even salty winter tyres. It is difficult to control porcupines. So like many rodents they virtually can destroy their surrounding. Differ-
ently to other rodents these porcupines only have 2-3 offspring, which are
breastfeed for 6 weeks. The body is covered with up to 20.000 quills, growing
from porcupine's back and sides and, in some species, from its head and tail.
The quills have needle-sharp ends containing hundreds of barbs. The quills of
Sphingurus have rings and are thinner than other porcupines'. Quills are up to
30 cm long; the colour is black and white. Skin muscles can erect them. Newborn porcupines' quills are elastic. They easily can loose them when they are
anxious or excited. There you can see kind of a lack in their defence mechanism: rebuilding those quills needs an awful lot of time; so loosing them means
loosing a part of their defence mechanism. They cannot touch each other and
warming each other is impossible without being hurt. Birds of prey become
their enemies. These animals possess a very strong and continued growth of
teeth. In nature normally they die before one can experience this pathology, as
they usually get killed by other animals when they grow old.

Sphingurus is exactly the contrary of a courageous animal. He frightens easily
like a rabbit. The porcupine looses his quills when someone gets closer, spasms
"make the quills fall out". Loss not caused by injury, but by anxiety. They can
easily die from a heart attack, just because they are so frightful

As rodents they are shy animals, live on trees, but over defensive still with thrills.
After an attack they could kill other animals. Because of spasms of the skin
muscles it loses his thrills and by accident other animals can earnestly be
wounded

Traditional use

In Brazil's traditional medicine quill powder is used against baldness, because
of the substance's composition.
People of the Indies liked to cook the animal. They used to dig a hole, cook it
over hot stones, then they skinned and ate it.

Proving

Why did it come to Mure´s mind to prove this remedy? Surely because of its
resemblance to easy loss of hair. We don't know exactly which kind of remedy

he used, because in his work he gave a description of an animal, which most probably is the described kind of porcupine above, the Sphingurus matini.

Authority. Mure, Pathol. Bresil. p.274. J.V. Martins took a dose of the 3d attenuation

Mind
Inconsistent and capricious mood (sixth day)
No inclination to work in the evening (first day)
Strong inclination to write in the morning, ceasing after breakfast (third day)

Head
Dizziness in the back of the head, when writing (third day)
Very heavy head, from 10 to 11a.m. (third day)
After breakfast drilling pain right through the skull's bones (second day)
Drilling pain through the skull-bones (fourth day)
Lancing pain on the left side of the head, through the skull-bones; inability to move the head for three minutes (fourth day)
Pain in one-half of the head (second day).
Slight prickling on the vertex from time to time, especially on the right side (third day)

Eye
Eyes fill with tears (fifth day)

Ear
Sharp pain from the left ear down to the jaw, for two minutes (fifth day)
Noise in the ears (second day)
Whizzing and humming from the left ear to the back of the head (third day)
Whizzing in the ears continues (third day)
Roaring in the ears, like a distant hurricane (third day).
Deafness in the left ear, as if blocked (sixth day)

Face
Pain in the right sigma (second day)
Long-lasting prickling in the sigma (third day)
Painful sensation in the jaw when articulating (third day)

Mouth
Bleeding of the gums (second day)

The toothache becomes obstinate (second day)
Pain in the first incisor tooth (second day)
Bitterness in mouth and throat, with salty taste (third day)

Stomach
Great appetite (fifth day)
Nausea at the sight of food (immediately), (first day).
Nausea with pain piercing through to the back.
Passing pains in toes, right temple, and one of the right canine teeth (second day)

All pain wares off after dinner (second day)
Aggravation when lying down, and improvement when walking in fresh air

Skin
Abundant desquamation in the regions of whiskers and chin (third day)
Itching all over, bleeding after scratching (sixth day)
Pubis itches considerably, after having tea (fourth day)

Sleep
Great drowsiness after dinner (first day)
Drowsy all day long (fourth day)
Drowsiness (fifth day)
Great tendency to yawn, with flow of saliva (fifth day)
Quiet sleep with cheerful dreams; morning, dreams about a multitude of insects, and a serpent which is very difficult to kill (third day)
Awaking early (second day)
Cheerful and quiet dreams (second day)
Cheerful dreams, at night (fifth day)

Fever
Chills from time to time (fifth day)
Trembling (horror) and chattering of teeth (second day)
Heat and numbness in the feet (fifth day)

Conditions
Aggravation
(When lying down), of symptoms.
(When stooping), pain in urethra.

Amelioration

(Walking in open air), of symptoms

(Motion), pain in arm

Case 1: Carmela, a nice woman aged 34

Rather timid, with an alarmed and embarrassed air about her, easily flushing. Over suspicious, but not that aggressive as Equisetum. Very shy person, difficult to talk about herself, especially before a man, difficult to show who she is. She lost lots of hair, is nearly bold. Different hormonal problems, many treatments without success. She was not so angry with the lots of wrong treatment, appreciated that the doctor tried to do something for her. In a certain moment he was in panic, shooting one remedy every week instead of telling he did not know what to do. So she was disappointed.

*** 'I'm well in general but what's bothering me is that I've lost so much hair, a really incredible amount. Nothing has helped at all, I've even been to a dermatologist, but nothing has helped. I didn't take any of the medications they gave me at the hospital because I'd rather have my liver than my hair and I've already taken so much medication in the past for my headaches that…

I was also treated homoeopathically. It helped for other things, but not for my hair. But then I didn't feel comfortable about the treatment any more because he always insisted on giving me the same remedy and I was always the same. He seemed a bit crazy about this remedy… he was giving it to me once a week and then I realised that he didn't understand me.

??- The hair loss has been a constant and unstoppable process. It became very sparse, especially at the front. I was told it was *androgenetic alopecia* and that I shouldn't have false hopes. I'm not so hopeful, but on the other hand, I'm ALMOST MORE ENRAGED AT NOT KNOWING THE REASON for why my hair is falling out.

I HAVE TO UNDERSTAND THINGS… IT'S IN MY DNA… OTHERWISE I FLIP OUT… I can't accept that things can happen to me, which I don't understand…

??- I have a weak heart, I take fright easily, and if something happens that I didn't foresee then I get even more frightened…

??- If something happens that I foresaw and I can understand it, then I get frightened and that's all... but my health doesn't suffer for it... and I don't lose my hair because of it.

??- I have had several tests, and they have proved inconclusive. But I've noticed that my nails have got into a really bad state, they're weak and grooved, so I've been taking mineral supplements for years...

??- They're very weak, and they bend. They've got ridges in them lengthways and they exfoliate.

??- I've never had strong nails, and for the last few years even my toenails have been weak. My skin isn't very good either; I think there's a problem with my "bark" in general.

** My digestion is slow and difficult, and I get rather tired. The tiredness affects my eyes especially. My eyesight has got worse and it feels like there are little needles in my eyes, and my head always feels very itchy. I had headaches for years and I think it's all due to tiredness and stress...

??- I mean that when too much stress builds up my system packs up... My digestion is the most recent thing... I started to have pains that also felt like thorns, a bit like with my eyes... and I also had cramps and a feeling of nausea which made me feel disgusted even just thinking about food...

Then this trouble with my head... I've had it for years. I was told I suffer from musculotensive headaches... WHAT IT MEANS IS THAT MY NECK IS ALMOST ALWAYS HARD AND TENSE.

When it happens it's... as though something was walking on your head, and sometimes I feel it in my face or in my hands or my belly and ALL I HAVE TO DO IS STROKE MY HAND OVER IT AND IT GOES... I also felt it years ago, and when I had any emotions, it was like a stroking feeling I felt in my face and then in my solar plexus... a shiver... I immediately get a lot of goose bumps on my head. Sometimes it doesn't take much, if something moves me or touches me emotionally I get a physical sensation of it...

??- What I meant is that I run my hand over it, and the feeling goes, but not the headache that comes on afterwards.

In the past I had to have very intensive treatment from a neurologist because I was suffering from trigeminal neuralgia and it was a disaster...

The only good thing about these pains is those years ago I suffered from a problem that I considered to be the opposite of what I have now. But they told me that on the contrary it was the same thing. ??- I had some facial hair, kind of like a beard, and a bit of a moustache… When I say it like that it sounds almost comic, but it wasn't in the least. It wasn't terrible… it's not very esthetic looking in a woman.

After I had the neuralgia, or after they gave me all that medication, the hair on my face started to disappear slowly… But it seems now I'm losing other hair which I would rather keep…'

*** 'Another big problem I have is that I often feel a knot in my throat… A while ago I used to feel this knot in my throat a lot, and if I squeezed it, it felt like someone was strangling me… As if someone was squeezing me… my throat feels squeezed. It happens if I'm agitated, or even for no apparent reason at all, though it's less now… Or if I'm feeling anxious, that can spark it off…'

??- *** 'It started after the divorce, because so many things were going wrong, not only from the point of view of the relationship. I had to rebuild EVERYTHING from scratch. It was difficult and it took a long time… I had to sort out so many things, even problems with my work.

??- I HAD TO GO ON A SURVIVAL COURSE. ALL OF A SUDDEN I FOUND MYSELF WITHOUT A PENNY, I HAD A DAUGHTER AND WAS OUT OF WORK… I thought I was with a certain kind of man and then he turned out to be completely different… I stopped eating and I weighed 49 kg, but I had a lot of energy, and I even did things at work just for the pleasure of it and not just to get by. But I had to think about my daughter. ??- She was only five years old.

UP TILL THEN I HAD ONLY EVER COUNTED ON MY HUSBAND BUT I NEVER REALLY TRUSTED HIM. I THOUGHT IT WAS ME THAT HAD ALL THE PROBLEMS AND THAT I COULDN'T BE EASY-GOING. INSTEAD IT WAS JUST BECAUSE I AM SURE THAT EVEN THEN I FELT THAT SOMETHING WASN'T QUITE RIGHT, SOMETHING WHICH WAS NEVER GOING TO WORK PROPERLY. I DISCOVERED ONE FINE DAY THAT HE WAS BETRAYING ME – WITH ANOTHER MAN….

I went to pieces; I could scarcely remember my own name (cries). It was useful in the sense that I found in myself qualities that I never knew I had… THE ABILITY TO DO THINGS. PLUS IT WAS A GOOD LESSON IN AWARENESS. It was a positive thing to happen in my life.

??- I wasn't aware and I felt fragile and weak and helpless, and I always needed the support of someone else… BUT TO BE HONEST I NEVER BELIEVED IN IT, NOT EVEN FROM MY PARENTS.

YOU CAN NEVER TRUST MEN.

Even paying the electricity bill was a problem for me... It taught me to evaluate things better and to trust my intuition and myself.'

??- ** 'OBVIOUSLY NOT, I would have fallen back into relying on someone else and blending in with them. I did have a strong desire to have another relationship, but I had some that didn't affect me for better or worse...

I had one relationship that lasted three years, but I finished it a few months ago. I USED TO BE HARD AND UNYIELDING, SOMEONE FOR WHOM THINGS WERE ALWAYS BLACK OR WHITE. But recently I've been more adaptable, and that is unusual for me.'

??- ** 'Three years ago I found the strength to decide to open a shop all by myself. I was very scared to launch myself into this, but I was always the manager in the shops I worked in. After the huge trauma of being abandoned it was good for me, and I went on a refresher course and retook my diploma...'

??- ** 'I often dream of famous people in normal situations in my life... ??- The Pope was one of the most recent ones, and the Minister of Health and the Prime Minister... in normal situations.

Discussion of the case:

Androgenetic alopecia, worse frontal

Weak nails, bending, rigid

Tired from stress

Digestion slow and difficult, pain like thorns and nausea in stomach, disgusting food

Eyesight <, like little needles in my eyes

Headaches, neck hard and tense, as if something was walking in my head, emotion = stroking feeling in face and solar plexus

Physical sensation when anything happens

Trigeminal neuralgia

Knot in throat, as if someone would strangling her, < with agitation

Dependent in the relationship, outside independent

Suspiciousness

No physical weakness as the other Silicas

More a change of sex, competition with another man male habit - loss of hair

Years ago facial hairs like a beard; skin problems.

Therapy Sphingurus Q1

<u>Follow up:</u>

She got headache with cervical pain and burning in urinal tract after 7 days.
For two months hair grows, then stopped. With Q3 hair growing again.
5 months later: Hair more and stronger and presented in a more feminine way.

"It feels as if my head was connected with my body in a different way. I am easily moved, I can weep now, and inside I feel much more sure. Before I never was allowed to show my emotions. After my divorce I became as thick as a piece of a horn, who's only right of existence was to keep people away from me.

Dreams of famous people

With such a sense of disgust and despise towards them. Even they are not able to do their own job. They feel so important, but they do the same stupid mistakes as anybody whom I could meet in the street. They lead wars, destroy the environment ... They should be impaled as the old Muslims did this. I had to build them up in my mind as idealistic persons, but now I see they cannot even stand on their own feet.

Desire to write

I wrote in my diary just a lot of bad words against others, slander... Just to keep these things far away from me. It is a kind of revenche that could be written only in my diary. A friend of mine who is a teacher said when reading this that her pupils can write much better than I can."

She is less chilly, has a different perception of her entire body, likes to buy new clothes, and wants to be more interesting for someone else. "I would like to trust in someone, I never could before."

Neuralgia, piercing pains

After 4 months – Herpes, trigeminus left side, which broke out when she was at the seaside with a friend, after 10days.

"We both were sure to have some fun, but then I had such a conflict: It was a pleasure to stay with him, but on the other side everything was hurting as if I would lie on a bed of thorns instead of a mattress. As if someone put some pins into my face. I had the same matter some years ago. I could have cut off my head. The neurologist behaved like a piece of bombastic shit."

"I did a photo when I was bald and showed to every man what I could become like."

Q5 cured the herpes after few days.

Case 2: Davide, 54 years

Herpes, neuralgia, stitching pains

Herpetic eruption
He comes because of a pain in his neck. Some time before he had intercostal neuralgia.
His red blood cell count too high
His mother died with 77 years because of a stroke

He is very shy and awkward.

"I feel like hovering in the air, I am out of my body. When I am talking it is as if another person talks, a state close to be drunk. This happens always in connection with problems in my work, then I do not feel my body, when I am under pressure."

"When I was younger I was very fond of writing."

I feel a strong pain in my chest, I am scared. Breathing is so painful but then I feel it also in other parts of my body. It started with an awful herpes, a very sudden stitching like a long arrow. I feel something piercing entering my body like voodoo witches.

I had an enlarged liver with a strong fever when I was 16 years, even my kidneys were infected and I was completely yellow.

I am scared of doctors, I cannot look at syringes. Tremendous fear, even now when they take blood. Appendectomy after fever that he had for a long time. The operation was a drama.

SPEECHLESS

I really never talked till the age of 13. I stopped talking after the age of 4 years and was completely silent for 9 years. I lived in a small village in Sicily. This time they brought to me my little cousin who was just born.

Image

People came to him to get advises; he was treated like a wise person.

When I went to school, the first 3 months I had very good marks, but then they threw me out. I studied philosophy at home on my own. With 13 I had to violate myself to do something. I took 3 shirts and 2 hats and I went to the coffee shop and asked for coffee.

Desire to write

In school I always used to write 2 pieces instead of one. From Sicily I changed to Milan and it took me two years to find some work. Everybody has his own world inside.

Estranged

When I talked I always had the impression I never belonged to this world.

To enter into a company I started working. At first I cleaned the floors. Later I made my own business, I became a manager for nearly bankrupt companies. Later I became vice major in my town. And I also won some prices in poetry. I was always afraid that other people could close me out."

Discussion:

I give you this extreme case of Sphingurus to show you how to work with this concept. What can you say about this extreme case?

Over-rational

Already at age 13 he speaks like an old wise man.

TIMIDITY

He always keeps the others in a save distance, "nolimetangere".

Every time he could not avoid coming nearer to other people in his work he left and went to another town and started from the scratch to work as an employee.

He published always under a pseudonym and did not want to join the writers club.

Extreme way to **restrict his environment**.

First not talking, then living in a strange environment.

Also his poetry was shrinked as much as it could be, like the juice of the juice of the juice. His concept of poetry was to put six words together - nothing more.

Extreme childhood, no mentioning of the parents, nor of his wife.

He likes being inside something bigger as the Russian puppets, one inside the other. He wears 3 shorts over each other, takes 3 companies over later, ...

He is working in one company after the other. He likes to be creative, one could be thinking of a drug remedy.

BEGINNING FROM THE SCRATCH

This is one of the most characteristic observation of Sphingurus cases. There was some kind of life, then something dramatic happened, then they change their entire life. As if they have to squeeze themselves into something totally new.

He could not remember which kind of experience he had at the age of four that made him change his life.

Itching, stinging

Herpetic eruptions

Follow up:

After Sphingurus he soon got an aggravation of his headache, a tension in his back. He decided to change his work; he quit his well-paid and well-considered job, gave away all his money for benefit and remained with very little money. He decided to go to work in a factory as a normal employee. He went away from Milan to another town, not telling people who he was. Little by little his physical symptoms improved completely, tension in the neck >>.

Two years after Sphingurus he started the first relationship of his life and he married some months later this woman who is even stranger than him. They also work together.

About the remedy:

We have little information in the repertory and most of the symptoms of Sphingurus erroneously came up under Spigelia. Out of a number of eighty-nine symptoms Sphingurus has sixty in common with Silica e.g. dreams animals, insects, snakes, capriciousness, indolence evening, mood changeable, aversion to work, talks embarrassed, vertigo in occipital.

Pain is perceived as shooting or digging, even stitching, and neuralgic. The clear symptoms of Sphingurus are more kind of a repeated prickling, a feeling of something injuring like a needle, the experience of being penetrated in some way. This could also be the description of a neuralgic pain. It was commonly used for neuralgic pains in the chest or in the face, whenever the pain was needle-like.

Timidity: another interesting matter is stammering, which usually you find under "larynx" or "mouth", but here very clearly is a mind symptom. M. Mangialavori reports three cases of this kind, more a problem of timidity, like people who are very shy, easily frightened when confronted with another person, which is unlike the stammering in remedies like *Agaricus*.

Sphingurus has only few mind symptoms:

Capriciousness: they never are happy with what they are doing. They want to know exactly how this toy is working. As soon as this matter is understood they throw it away. They are over-rational – found in two cases of Sphingurus children. Over precision (like Silica people). Obsessive in what they are doing.

Indolence, aversion to work

Desire to write.

Dreams of famous people

The meaning of the dreams could be that they really feel very tiny. Then these famous people are perceived as shit, probably as they are also just human. When progressing in their therapy the patients understand that they are not so high above everything, but normal people with normal mistakes.

Dreams snakes: All the remedies that have a relationship to snakes could have a connection to the evil. I think for Sphingurus it is something snaky that could violate your inner space in a special way they cannot see, they cannot perceive. It is a symbol of something very small that could enter and is impossible to be controlled. The meaning of snakes in Silica, Sphingurus, and Bambusa too, is not similar to sexual symbols in other remedies. In my experience it is not of such importance. Silica-likes are not the first group of remedies I would think of concerning this topic. It is such a complex symptomatology, this fear of snakes.

DD drugs:

If I had followed him into his delusions, I would have prescribed a drug. But his way of behaviour is not like a drug. Stressing himself to be able to grow, I never saw in drugs. These patients here are much more grounded. His seemingly out of body experience is a deep in body feeling, a mentally moving in and in and in. He has an over rational attitude to get an explanation about what happens in the world. It is more a look into the mirror, to realise what is right and wrong. This over analytical point of view is typical for Sphingurus. At the same time intuition can be well expressed, together with this over rational attitude. But on the other side it is impossible to integrate any kind of feeling.

This patient of case 2 was as sensitive as he was over rational. He stopped talking, withdrew from his surroundings, and then used his rational approach. He could think so rational and analytical, that, coming from a little village in Sicily, without studying, he became a big manager. Just because he had such a powerful ability to analyse what is here and there. He is able to understand deeply how things work, to cut mentally everything into pieces.

All the Sphingurus patients I really had to squeeze a lot to get some information! It is difficult to understand them deeply, because I was not able to get in good contact with them, it is even more difficult than with Kali-sil. I just can tell you the phenomena. The ability, the skills to push yourself and to react, to squeeze yourself into something completely different than before is very special for them.

What all my three adult Sphingurus cases had in common was first of all that I was really sure that they were Silica cases, but Silica did not work. They where very shy persons, had a lot of problems of anticipation, before examinations etc. They where complaining about offensive perspiration and they easily perspired, mostly when they where excited. One of them started to loose hair after a serious stress and the three of them had to quit their work because it was too stressful for them. Like in Silica they where very professional, very precise and wanted to be recognised from the others. In the moment of performance they start to perspire very intensely, from a longer stress they develop a kind of greasy skin (goose flesh) and lose their hair.

One had an ulcer in the stomach and he was complaining about severe stitching pains. He said, my doctor understood immediately that it was an ulcer because I was able to say exactly on which point I had the pain. It was like an arrow in my stomach and because of this pain I could not continue to eat. His preferred food was anything basic, he very fond of nuts and other dry fruits.

At that time I did not know that Sphingurus was a rodent and I searched in different directions to find out the remedy for this seemingly clear Silica case. I tried different potencies, gave him something more specific for the stomach without good result. So one day, looking again to the symptoms I had the idea to consider Sphingurus. I considered this also because of another possible relationship. You know how much Sphingurus is related to Silica? They need to have a special food that contains a lot of silica, especially something from the bark of the trees. As I told you it is a serious problem when they loose their quills because they have to build this prickle new. First it is absolutely elastic. When it becomes thick and rigid – like in bamboo – this is due to the content of silica. So I tried to prescribe Sphingurus. Besides I could not observe any other good symptom. It was a very close person, very reserved, very shy, and not able to express anything. His father has a small business, but he was not able to work with his father because he said he could only work on his own. This is all I was able to find out. Sphingurus brought a very good result. I could not observe a growing of the hair, but no more hair loss - alopecia areata- and the pain in the stomach was much better in a short time. It worked even a lot on the skin, he lost his gooseflesh reaction. I saw him after more then one year. After feeling better – as typical for Silica patients- he escaped as quickly from the doctor as he could. He came because of a relapse of his stomach pain, which manifested when he was invited by his priest to organise a celebration in the church. There his lady was working, teaching about catechisms. He had had this relationship for one year till she decided to become a nun. He had a serious collapse, for him it was a huge stress, because they had talked about marriage seriously, also already with her family. I think she did not have any desires and he was so depressed that in this situation he tried to ask something about sex. Up to then his sexual life for me was an absolutely closed box. Besides his stomach pain he had also constipation and the skin problem with the gooseflesh started again. Before coming to me he went to different healers to have some magic treatment done, but they did not have any result. When he came to me he mainly complained about this stitching pain. After Sphingurus he was much better in a short time. So, this is why I wanted to present something about Sphingurus, because it is very unknown.

Differential diagnosis of ***Natrums and Silicas*** concerning difficulties in communicating:

Generally Natrums also use the strategy to make you move for them, a way of letting others take care for you, of showing that you are different and stubborn, which, when you consider it, is a way to be seductive really. In Silica the lack of communication does not arise because they want other people to be closer to them; they are anxious in some way, they think that other people could persecute them. So in Silica like remedies the relationship with others is always kind of a defensive situation, also in Sphingurus. Symbolically talking, even the energy they use to defend themselves is a lot of energy. So for the Natrums it is important to demonstrate that normally you want others to come to you, in Silica it is really difficult to stand a relationship, to be able to confront; whenever you have to face a relationship it is riskfull, because the other person could take profit of you. In these cases the Silica group reacts like a baseball, bouncing back and forth, being touched by an attack or a discussion, but instantly taking off to another direction without becoming emotionally involved. So, after a short contact/impact, they avoid to discuss what's really going on, without being untouchable. They don't use such specific strategies. It is common for them to have a bad relation with their doctor: as soon as you have cured them they don't like to return. Normally they are not able to work by themselves, you can find an imbalance of wanting to do something very well and not wanting to have any responsibility.

Two cases of M. Mangialavori reported a stitching pain in the chest and eruptions; both of them had red spots with many of the common symptoms of Silica. They started to loose their hair when they where quite young and one of them had an alopecia.

Remarkable difference to **Baryta** in general:

In all the Barytas, like in Calciums, the need of getting really strong support is very prominent A Baryta child clings to its mother - You can't really say this for the Silica group; there you find some kind of fanaticism, which to my mind is more a matter of suspicion than of real religiosity, a desperate attempt to get the support you never had in your life. So instead of a real relationship you create fantastic relationships; which is more often represented in Equisetum, than in Sphingurus.

Summary of Sphingurus themes

Unreliable support
Image
TIMIDITY
SPASM – poor defence
RESTRICTED ENVIRONMENT, extreme withdrawal, estranged from environment
Over rational, deep understanding, estranged from emotions
Stiffness
Slow reaction
BEGINNING FROM THE SCRATCH

ALOPECIA

Pain piercing/stitching/neuralgic/shooting/prickling
Hair, nails, skin, digestion
CERVICAL REGION; THYREOID; THROAT, SPEECHLESS, stammering
Desire writing
Dreams important people
Snakes
Chill

HECLA LAVA

Substance:

In Hecla lava we have to consider very different qualities in comparison what we have seen until now because even if Hecla lava is so full of silica it must be different. It is a complicated substance and we have the ash of it, the blackish-brown ash of Monte Hecla in Island.

In a very basic point of view, considering the well known side, we have many symptoms in common with Silica; all the symptoms we have seen about suppuration, difficult healing, bone symptoms, abscesses, neuralgia in the face. But Hekla contains many substances, not only silica. It is also full of sulphur, and is also called "cold sulphur".

Discussion of homeopathic symptoms and themes:

In common with Silica is this tendency towards easy infection, normally a result of penetration. It covers a special kind of injury where the wound does not receive oxygen; it is not a bleeding kind of injury.

A special symptom of Hekla is that the person does not seem to take care of his symptomatology. As Bambusa they want to show I am resistant, but different from Bambusa they are very volcanic and creative personalities, but also very good in logic. Their creativity is developed in a very selected, specific field, where they perform, get their attention in society and thus can find their place in society, which will always be a chief position. So they can overcome their lack of self-confidence, they are a genius in their field and workaholics, which is their excuse not to have a normal contact with other people. This is their strategy to receive attention and to be loved by other people, to be well considered. They seek for appreciation very much.

M. Mangialavori: I have three cases where I prescribed with very good results Hecla lava for osteomyelitis, where these persons came to see me in a bad state, not taking care at all what they had. Even if it was a really painful situation, as an osteomyelitis usually is, they seemed to think about it only when the doctor said, you know it's possible that you will loose this toe e.g. I had the very strong impression that they wanted to show their strength, that they are not so easy to attack by an illness. One patient is an animator in a tourist village, but out of his job he is a very hidden personality, cannot entertain spontaneously, only perform it as a mask. All Hekla patients appear quite mechanical personalities to me. They are very kind people; never have discussions or quarrels with anybody. In public they appear sure, self-confident, get attention, show how professional they are. Private they are shy, blushing easily and grinding their teeth during sleep like Silica. In public they show only their surface as also *Sulphur, Selen, Petroleum, Palladium* do. Privately they like to be in nature and especially near the water. They can be sailors and like to swim.

The sickness is then like an inner explosion, a destructive reaction. Also on the mental level we have after a long time a sudden outburst and then the relationship is over. After that they experience a strong sense of guilt and feel that everything is their fault. As in the volcanoes we have long quiet periods, then there is an eruption and then it is over forever. So they always remain alone. With forty years they have a cemetery of relationships. To be able to stay in a relationship they need a very high position. Their sense of duty is higher than in *Aurum*. Underneath there is a very poor sense of self-confidence because it was never estimated what they did.

The pathologies are long and deep and seem to start suddenly. But they only realise the situation suddenly when it is already there for a long time.

You can see that the main symptoms are strongly affecting the male side. Most of the pains are sore, bruised, pain during urination.

There are many spine problems and Hekla is a great remedy for the feeling that the spine is too weak - also without neuralgia.

Summary of Themes

weak structure
unreliable support
stiffness/rigidity/image – pretended sociability
restricted environment/withdrawal/hold in
SUDDEN EXPLOSION

Inner resistance/stubbornness
Slowness in development, chronic suppurative processes, slow healing process

chilly
WATER

perspiration (foot, head)
restlessness
sensitive to noise
aversion to milk, mother's milk, milk agg.
chronic suppurative processes
hair, nails, bones, epidermis, mucous membranes

So we find an inflexible, rigid, stubborn person who is fixed to a certain image, which he wants to fulfil. His opinion is fixed, he has fixed ideas, thinks he is accepted when he fulfils a fixed, perfect image. It is very important what others think about him - "yielding aspect", "lack of self-confidence"- which picture they have from him and he fulfils it in a very stubborn rigid way. He has to defend his ideas, his picture -"intolerance of contradiction"- The main compound Silica is mostly found in human structures, which are needed for defence (nails, epidermis, teeth, bones).

Other opinions, ideas, changing systems, are experienced as a threaten to his person. His "digital" approach to life (perfect, rigid, reproducing), like computers (Silica as a basic element of semiconductors, chips etc.) does not allow an "analogue", creative, inventing way of being. His seemingly creative side is a role, wanting to be creative. Hekla, like Silica, can just break, not bend, like glass. (breaking/splitting symptoms, like splitting nails, delusion is divided in two, left side does not belong to her.

PARASITES

CIMEX LECTULARIUS

Latin: acanthia lectularia, cimex lectularius
English: Bed bug,
German: Bettwanze

Classification:

Arthropodes, Insects, (hexapoda), Rhynchota /Hemipterateroptera, Gymnocerata

Description

The name Cimex micis is Latin for "stinking like a mouse". In a figurative way in Italian the name is used for someone who is malicious, dirty, repellent and greedy for money. The "cimices" or in German "Wanze" is a kind of microphone that you can hide easily.

Bugs live with men or mammals. They can be found living behind the wallpaper. They also climb up on the ceiling and drop down on the host. The mostly affected beside men are birds and bats. They suck their host's blood during night changing colour when sucking the blood.

The adult bedbug is flat and has a more or less oval shape. It is approx. 5 mm long and 3 mm wide. The body is covered with fine, short hair and is usually brown. Shortly after drinking blood, however, it is reddish, or dark red to violet, if the stomach still contains blood from a previous meal. When bedbugs need blood, they are as thin as paper, but after a generous meal, they are much fatter and can be even spherical. They have lost the ability to fly; in fact, all they have left are a few rudimentary stumps on the middle segment of the chest area. (Vermeulen).

There is a marked inability to adapt to changes of temperatures. When the temperature is less than 16° C, bugs don't eat anymore. As with most of the blood sucking parasites, they can fast for a long time. When they do eat, they gain six times their bodyweight within ten minutes.

Cimex finds his host by his smell and warmth. Interestingly, the insects can produce an ugly smell. They also tend to gather in places where their own sorts are already present. They are attracted by the smell of glandular discharges and secretion of their fellows. As is the case with many bugs, they emit a penetrating odour. They shun light completely.

Evolutionarily, they have a relationship to bats. Originally they had wings but have now lost their abilities to fly. There are five stages of development, and a blood meal is required in each. The female lays two or three eggs a day, up to a total of 150 to 200. The eggs are dropped into cracks and crevices and firmly attached using a glue-like substance. In the case of a temperature of 28° C, the eggs hatch after five or six days. (Vermeulen) The symptoms after their bites or stings are most prominent in the liver and digestion systems, including haemorrhoids, a malaria-type fever may appear, with alternation of heat and chill while the person is thirsty. There are often gastric headaches after drinking. The stinging is painful, and unfortunately for the host, if they don't sting, they cannot eat. Laboratory studies have shown that a bedbug refuses to suck food that is otherwise suitable if there is no skin, which it can first puncture. So the idea of penetration is very important. It is suspected that they transmit several diseases. The saliva contains histamine-like substances. The saliva also contains substances that ensure that the host's blood doesn't clot.

From "Natural History of Animals" (Reference Works)
A small family of vampire insects whose love for the close society of humans during the hours of darkness is not requited. The common bed bug is by far the best-known and most abundant species, and the descriptive material, which follows, applies to it. The rare, blind, wingless bat parasites of the family Polyctenidae are close relatives of the bed bugs.

Adults: Flat, wingless, hairy with 4-segmented antennae of which the last 2 segments are much more slender than the others. The head, with conspicuous protruding eyes, is sunken in a wide notch in the rim of the first thoracic segment; there are no ocelli. During the day bed bugs hide under mattresses, behind loosened wallpaper, baseboards, and in other dark crevices. They may exist without feeding for a year or so under otherwise favourable conditions. Besides man, bed bugs feed upon various rodents, cattle and horses, and poultry. The elongate, white eggs 1/32 inch long, with little raised cap at one end, are glued a few at a time to the surfaces of the hiding places. "Bed bug odour" is due to the oily secretion from a pair of glands, which open on the underside of the third thoracic segment.

Young: Quite similar to the adults and likewise bloodsucking. Development from egg to adult requires 4 to 6 weeks; there are 5 nymphet stages.

Importance: The common bed bug is not a proven disease carrier; its bite, how-ever, is in many instances followed by intense itching, swelling, and reddening of the skin. A southwestern species of another genus attacks poultry and is oc-casionally a nuisance in houses. Species of still other genera feed on swallows, martins, and chimney swifts; they live in the nests over winter, awaiting the spring return of the migrants. Bats are attacked by several cimices.

The English names for the common bedbug (Cimex lectularius) were "chinches," "wall-louse" and just plain "bug." "Bug" is a Celtic word signifying a ghost or goblin, probably because the Celts considered bedbug's terrors of the night. This family of blood-sucking bugs contains not over twenty species in the world, eight of which are recorded from North America. The young, immedi-ately upon hatching, look like smaller editions of their parents. Both young and adult bedbugs feed by sucking blood. At no stage of life do they have wings. To emphasize their ability to get where there is plenty of food the following verse is widely quoted:

> The June bug hath a gaudy wing,
> The lightning bug a flame,
> The bedbug hath no wings at all
> But he gets there just the same.

Traditional use:

Dioskorides says that 7 bugs eaten before the onset of malaria quartana can be helpful and also that bugs triturated and inserted into the urethra can cure in-flammations and reduce spasm of urethra Bedbugs have in the past been rec-ommended for a great variety of ailments. As an ointment for the eyes, crushed bedbugs mixed with salt and human milk were used. In powdered from they were believed to cure all fevers. For hysteria they were given internally and just the smell of them was considered sufficient to relieve those under hysterical suffocation. Eating seven bedbugs mixed with beans was believed to help those suffering with quartana plague, provided the eating was done before the onset of the attack, and even at the present time in certain areas of Ohio this same mixture is considered good as a cure for chills and fever. At one time bedbugs were also thought to be especially good as neutralizers of serpent venom, that of asps in particular, as well as a useful preventative against all other kinds of poisons.

Hahnemann (Apothekerlexikon):
"This.... incredibly stinking insect has been used in former times as a disgusting diuretic remedy and also (irrationally) to abort the afterbirth and it has been used against quartana fever. You could even make people regain their consciousness after fainting by the stinking odour of the smashed bugs."
The odour results from the secretion of glands on the ventral metathorax of the bugs.

Bedbugs have in the past been recommended for a great variety of ailments. As an ointment for the eyes, crushed bedbugs mixed with salt and human milk were used. In powdered from they were believed to cure all fevers. For hysteria they were given internally and just the smell of them was considered sufficient to relieve those under hysterical suffocation. Eating seven bedbugs mixed with beans was believed to help those suffering with quartan plague, provided the eating was done before the onset of the attack, and even at the present time in certain areas of Ohio this same mixture is considered good as a cure for chills and fever. At one time bedbugs were also thought to be especially good as neutralizers of serpent venom, that of asps in particular, as well as a useful preventative against all other kinds of poisons.

CIMEX in Homeopathy:

The original proving

of cimex lectularius was performed by W.Whale, M.D. from Rome, one of Hahnemann's earliest disciples. Only three provers were participating.
The remedy is made from whole insect.
Main symptoms:

- Weariness
- Inclination to stretch as if tendons were contracted (especially hamstrings)
Feels he cannot run fast enough
Extremities: as if too short, cannot move as they would like
- Stiffness
- Delusion: has to crawl together and make himself as small as possible
Sense of persecution, needs to hide
- Drinks greedily and afterwards there is nausea
- Every symptom worse after drinking
- Eating and drinking seem unpleasant
- Enormous appetite
- Tendency to fill the stomach
- It is better to have thirst than move to get something to drink
- Tearing pains
- Perceiption of pain is exaggerated
- Extreme descriptions
- Hysterical persons who perceive pains strongly - (all insects, Canth, Apis, Vespa)
- Destructiveness: not only in words, similar to cantharis, tears things to pieces
- Kids find pleasure in being offensive and destroying to show their power
- Most sensations are stitching, stinging, penetrating
- Connection between burning and stitching/stinging, gives a very irritated picture

CASE, 54 year old man

The patient is a very unpleasant person. He is the owner of a nightclub, known because he was in prison several times for cocaine possession. He is in the business of trading of cars coming from abroad. The origins of the cars often were not so clear because they might be stolen cars. He is not at all adversely affected by having such an awful fame.
He is very irritable with no sense of humour. When I tried to make some joke, he would not react at all. He only spoke short sentences with a rough, abrupt and direct way of talking. He was very impolite, awful language and crude sex jokes. He only is loudly laughing about his own jokes and as a result a great sense of compassion woke in me. I thought, what a poor person. He was dressed

with an open shirt, showing a bush of hair coming out, some tons of golden chains around his neck and an enormous Rolex on his wrist. While talking he was often showing a disgusted expression in his face, and strongly macho. Before he came we had some discussion and he was lamenting and complaining that he wanted to come immediately. When I told him that wasn't possible he offered to pay more.

"I can say I have had every possible treatment. I have such a headache, that it drives me crazy. I don't know what to do. Please help me! I have been suffering from it for years. My head is bursting. It is here in my forehead. It is as if my brain would escape. I have also suffered for years from sinusitis but this is different. This piece of shit in the hospital (meaning the doctor) they are so obstinate in prescribing treatment for my sinusitis. I have broken my testicles with this kind of rubbish. I am really suffering. Give me something very strong. I cannot take it anymore."

Can you describe the pain?

"It is an awful, tremendous pain."

When did it start?

"It started after a strong flu with a very high fever. There started this kind of torture. Until four years ago, I had nothing. Then I went to Tanzania for vacation. I had to go back, because I got malaria, in spite of all the medication that I took. I destroyed my liver taking the drugs and then I still had malaria. Such a piece of shit. I would like to break my head on the wall. The other day I destroyed a complete set of dishes, then I felt better."

Which kind of problem do you have in your digestion?

"My stomach is completely blocked and my bowels, too. I cannot even drink even if I perceive such dryness in my throat. I have the feeling of a piece of coal inside, a burning that I cannot describe. And then I have something on my tongue, a kind of dirty white stuff. I would like to drink liters of water and I don't drink only water but I take alcohol and sometimes some cocaine. I eat like a pig. The idea of having a snack doesn't exist. If I am hungry I have to eat and then after filling my stomach I can stay for hours without touching any food, even without drinking. I cannot eat like the homosexuals! (He means eating little and dandy like, dainty.) I have to eat a lot but meat is something that nobody can take away from my diet otherwise I can eat the one."

Any favourite food?

"Nothing that I prefer. I just eat, that's all. What is disgusting to me is water. It can take away my sense of thirst but the idea of drinking disgusts me."

Any other problems?

"The sinusitis, since I was a child. Once I destroyed the door of the fridge because of the strong pain. (He had to break something because of his irritation from the pain.)"

Do you remember something more about that time?

"I was continuously vomiting at that time. I had such dirtiness in my mouth and since then I had the feeling of something that is burning and cooking in my mouth. I could have eaten more, just to feel more calm but I cannot break something every time I am sick."

How is the pain?

"I had the feeling of a pick stung in my face and sometimes it was moving from my forehead to my vertex. It was a kind of bloody pain even in the root of my nose. It is hurting even now but not so strongly as before. Shit. When I am like this, my mouth and my tongue are burning. Sometimes I cannot even brush my teeth because of the pain. You can imagine the meat remaining between my teeth. My girlfriend says the odour from my mouth can kill a camel from 10 meters. But I don't care at all. I need not kiss anybody."

What do you mean?

"I have overcome that period of my life: the girlfriends, the kisses, going out for dinner, dancing, a lot of shit stuff. At the end you and she, too, know you are just going out to fuck. Now I arrive directly at that point with women, if they like it. (He talks about the position that he prefers in sex.) I like it like the animals and possibly using both entrances. (He says this in awful expressions.)"

Do you remember other problems?

"I did a lot of sports but I had to stop because of strong cramps. My muscles became so stiff but when young everything is so stiff! (He is implying that not only the muscles but also the cock.) I know the medicine for that! I was playing rugby and soccer, because I like to kick the ball and not only the ball! (He is implying he kicks people too.) I had to stop because I had this pain in my fingers and in my toes. I remember that my doctors gave me magnesium but it was a shit therapy. Now I have the same pain when I have headache and when I get a fever. This was the first symptom - the stiffness in my muscles."

About your sleep?

"My sleep is a shit, my life is a shit and this is why I sleep like shit. Once when I was not able to sleep I had a good fuck and with the discharge I could sleep very well. Now with all the coffee that I drink, it is bad. I tried to stop smoking and drinking coffee but it did not change."

Dream?

"I don't remember, and if I remember it is just shit."

What do you mean with all this shit?

"Once I used to dream about some cloacae that was full and I sensed just an awful smell that I could not stand. But it was the only place where I could hide and escape. (He was being pursued). I dreamed this for long time, but it was a real shit."

Relationship with women?

"My relationship with women doesn't exist, but that is OK. Sometimes I meet one with whom I have a good fuck. I have something else to think about. My business is the most important thing. I have two nightclubs and I am very busy."

With other people?

"It is a pleasure as long as there is a competition. If I am not the winner I am very angry. Everybody is stealing something from others and I steal what I can. This is my commitment and I learned that from people whom did other people train. I learned it in prison."

What do you mean?

"You know who taught me most in life? It was no priest, no doctor no shit psychologist. It was a guard in prison. He had seen so many people in his life, many more than any psychologist. Whenever he saw a person, after 30 seconds he was able to tell you all the details of that person. He never made a mistake. He had such a big, golden heart. He used to say that it is a law of nature. Even if we want to consider ourselves different from beasts, it is not true. People are killing people; even priests do what is important for them. The only difference is that I have the courage to tell it. If you behave like a nice person and not asking for more then there is a place for everybody in this world. That means that other people like me can have more than that. I am scratching like a leper. Anyway I scratch like someone who has to scratch. When I go to sleep I have to scratch my testicles until they hurt. My digestion is not so good. My bowels are not working. They told me it is just because I am very nervous. I even remember that they asked me to have an examination to measure my bowels. (That is what he understood.) I said yes, but then they put this awful stuff in my ass to check the pressure. They said it was too high! I would have liked to see the doctor's face if someone put that stuff in his ass if he had not clenched too. Even if my stools are not so hard I have severe constipation (It is because of the extreme contraction of his sphincter).

CASE, a stallion

The stallion has a very athletic body with many muscles. He is a tournament horse. Until now he had very good results. Recently he had serious character problems. The owner called some special trainers to help his mood. Unfortunately, at that moment they thought they would have to kill him because he was so violent. Everything started after a serious fever that arose after a competition. His groom kept him. Then all of a sudden he escaped from him and started to fight with another stallion. The two horses jumped out on to the competition field. In this kind of competition, the other stallion was faster and better. At the end he started to bite and kick until they were able to separate the two. He left the other horse severely hurt. After that suddenly he had stiffness in joints. His legs were very swollen, and there was titanic rigidity. They thought he had tetanus, but he had been vaccinated for that. The next day he had a very high fever. He refused to drink. He was very restless, always moving from the laying down position to standing up. When the fever was very high he bit everything, even the metal cup for his water. He tried to escape from the box by knocking his head against the wall. After two days of high fever he became much more violent. It was not easy to ride him. When riding him, he suddenly would go straight on to an obstacle or to the wall with the intention to hit and kill his rider. They tried to change his bit several times without any result. A second rider tried to train him. When the horse started to run downhill on a hill full of stones, the rider jumped off the horse to save himself. After that he had moments of fever that lasted for 36 or 48 hours during which the horse was even more terrible and violent. They had to put him in another box, because he destroyed his own wooden box. The only possibility to calm him down was by putting a blanket over him. This worked even though it was not cold at that time. His appetite and thirst were inconstant. Some days he would not touch any food and on other days he ate everything, even the bark off of trees. When he had fever he did not eat anything. They suspected a kind of worm or viral infection, but the owner did not want to spend money on more examinations. The stiffness, too, was very inconstant. Sometimes it was impossible for him to walk. He would overreact to any light stimulus with a kind of tension. His stool and urine were very offensive, which was new since he had been sick. When the fever was high he opened mouth and moved his tongue from side to side. His mouth was really hot inside, like a kind of glossitis. His urination was very inconstant. He could remain for hours without having stool or without urinating. His behaviour towards water changed. He didn't want to drink water with the other horses. He would only drink alone in his own box. Before he was able to jump across water but now he stopped. He absolutely refused to cross a river when alone. If competing with another horse, he always wanted to cross first. He always used to seek places in the shadow otherwise he could get very nervous in the sun. If they wanted to make him calm down they had to put a kind of mask over his eyes, so that he looked into the dark. He was much more libidinous than before. It was not possible to keep him quiet when a female horse was near. Often he used to stretch like a cat, which was very strange for a horse.

Cimex 10 M resolved the stallion's problems quickly so that he did not have to be killed.

Comments, considering the cases, differential-diagnostic aspects

The relation with water is very specific for Cimex.

Like Hirudo, Cimex shuns the light.

Unlike Hirudo, there is a lot of competition in Cimex.

The competitive side of the **Labiatae** is a much more creative one than in Cimex where the only purpose is to be the first. The Labiatae try to improve and build up something for others. In Cimex it is destruction, much more like **Mercurius** or **Syphilinum**. **Vespa** and **Apis** are competitive too. They are proud of their capacities in their work, there is a positive production. **Cantharis** also reach their goals. Cimex is similar but they don't seek a social position. They feel they are like poisonous animals so they want to distinguish themselves from the rest of the society. This distinction is underlined very much by them. Cimex is verbally aggressive to show their macho way. They need to demonstrate that they are able to penetrate another person's world.

Photophobia seems to be a common matter in many insects, like Cantharis or Apis. Fear of water is also a common insect characteristic, as in Cantharis or Coccinella septempunctata. Although insects are found anywhere from the South Pole to the North Pole, there is not one insect that lives in the water. Insects represent 70 % of the animals in the world, and two thirds of our planet is covered with water but no insect lives there. They can stay in damp environment but not in the water.

We must underline that there is a foxy, tricky part of the life of cimex.

Noble metals feel the task of doing something. *Niccolum* wants to appear as precious as gold, and is therefore very competitive. When Niccolum lose, they get a severe depression like the great fear of losing we see in Aurum. The desire to "fill up" in the parasites is in proportion to what they feel they are missing.

Insects need to work as little as possible for big results. Spiders work ten times as much. They need to be seen in their activities. Insects, however, might work in a hidden way. The important thing for them is to make money and to have results.

The spider's attitude is a demonstrative one, a kind of hysterical personality, in which he needs to show his activity even more than achieve results.

PEDICULUS HUMANUS CAPITIS

English: Head louse,
German: Menschenkopflaus

Classification

Arthropodes, Insectes, Phthiraptera, Anoplura, Pediculus humanus capitis

Description

Pediculus is a parasite affecting many different kinds of animals, especially the animals with hair or feathers. In Spanish, Greek, French and Italian, lice refer to persons who make a lot of money and show it in a haughty way.

NATURAL HISTORY of ANIMALS (Reference Works):

Like the adults and the young of other North American families of sucking lice, these bear a superficial resemblance to a crab when seen through a magnifying lens, owing to the strongly flattened body and the powerfully clawed, crab-like legs. This family is our most important one, containing parasites of the horse, hog, sheep, goat, dog, and of cattle and numerous wild rodents. All species are bloodsucking. The eggs, or nits, are glued to the hairs of the host. The young ones resemble the adults in appearance. There are usually 3 nymphet stages; metamorphosis is incomplete. The entire life cycles of these insects are completed upon the host animals. They are a source of much annoyance to the hosts and sometimes numerous enough to cause serious illness and death. The word "louse" is often applied to insects, which are not true lice, such as the book louse, the plant louse (the aphid), and the bark louse (the scale insect), and the bee louse (which is a fly). As a matter of fact, the term "louse" is often applied to animals that are not even insects, such as the wood louse (the sow bug or pill bug), and the fish louse. In this chapter we shall concern ourselves only with the true "blood-sucking" lice in this Order (Anoplura)-the lice that are parasitic on mammals-because they are the ones that may affect human beings. Lice are small insects, somewhat flattened in form, and like the fleas they are blood-sucking parasites that do not at any time possess wings. Their mouthparts are also of the piercing-sucking type. When the beak of a louse is not in use it is completely withdrawn into the head so that all one can usually see externally, through a microscope, is a fringe of minute teeth at the foremost part of the head. Lice have developed strong claws, situated at the end of the last joint of each of their six legs, which clasp hairs firmly, thus enabling them to maintain a hold on active animals. These claws are also used to hold on to seams of clothing usually the inside seams, in order to take advantage of human body warmth. The female louse "cements" her eggs, commonly called "nits," to the inner seams of woollen clothing and to the hair of man or other mammals. One female may lay an average of ten eggs a day for a period of from twenty to thirty days. The young become active as soon as they hatch, proceeding to suck blood with their unique mouthparts. The young resemble the adults in shape and form from the moment they hatch. Lice are highly specialized insects normally found on their preferred animal hosts. In other words, animal lice will usually be found only on certain animal hosts, while human body lice prefer and are invariably found on human beings. Lice are also very sensitive to what has been aptly called the climatic condition of the skin, its temperature and humidity, and prefer a temperature slightly lower than that of the body, which they ordinarily find by clinging to seams of clothing next to the body or to the hairs of mammals. If the body has a high fever, or if the body cools, as when death takes place, the lice will leave and seek another host. The species of lice infesting man are considered to be three in number: the head louse, the body louse, and the pubic or "crab" louse. They vary in colour from white to brown. When young and recently fed, the blood meal can be seen through the skin and they appear to be bright red. In military vocabulary they are then known as "red backs." As digestion takes place the blood becomes darker. They are then often called "black backs" or "grey backs." Because of these changes in coloration the same lice are often mistaken for different species. In soldier's slang in World War I all body lice were known as "cooties," but World War II made that term obsolete the modern version is "motorized dandruff!" Body lice and head lice can transfer from one person to another upon contact, and sitting next to an infested person in a train is a close enough contact for this transfer to take place. Normally, lice are rather slow-moving insects, but they are capable of moving with sufficient speed to give weight to the old saying: "You can't catch a louse with one finger." Lice undergo a metamorphosis according to the part of body where they are living. There are two kinds of animals: capitis and pubis. Pediculus corporis is longer and of light colour and it is able to live even in clothes especially woollen things. They stay during the day in the tissue and during night they sting and suck the blood. That results in a very strong itching, which seems to be the strongest among the animals. The tremendous itching often affects the whole body and not just what is affected by the bite. Secondary infections from scratching are common. Chicken, elephants, rhinoceros are infested and one is even a parasite of apis. Another one is affecting apples and spends its whole life in the body of one victim. (thus demonstrating affection and fidelity that has become rare among humans) It is not easy to get rid of the eggs. They are the most sensitive to light!

http://www.museums.org.za/bio/insects/lice/pediculus-capitis:

The eggs (or 'nits') of head lice are attached to hairs and the nymphs which hatch from them resemble the adults except being smaller. Depending on temperature, it takes 2-4 weeks for the eggs to hatch, the nymphs to pass through three moults and the adults to reach sexual maturity.

Treatment: There are three main approaches to treating head lice infestations.

Insecticide shampoo. Two main types of shampoos are available in South Africa. The cheaper (and most commonly used) of the two contains Gamma Benzine Hexachloride otherwise known as lindane. There have been a number of horror reports of lindane causing neurological problems and the National Pediculosis Association in the U.S.A. strongly recommends that it should not be used. If you do use a lindane-based shampoo, follow the instructions very carefully particularly with regard to how often you can apply it. The other shampoo, which is more expensive, contains permethrin, which has a much better safety record than lindane. Combing the hair with a louse comb is regarded as a very effective method but it takes time Plastic louse combs (which sometimes come with the shampoo you buy) are regarded as ineffective and a metal one should be used instead. Application of oils: There is good anecdotal evidence that application of certain long-chain oils to the hair is effective in removing lice infestations. Coconut oil or olive-oil-based shampoo (or bar soap or pure oils) is recommended in combination with combing. You can make up the following recipe: 30 ml olive oil, 20 drops of tea tree oil, 10 drops rosemary oil, 10 drops lavender oil and 10 drops lemon oil. With this recipe, first test that there is no skin reaction by applying a little of this solution to the inside of the elbow and wait a few hours to see if there is any adverse reaction. Apply this solution to the hair and leave it there for an hour, then shampoo (the shampoo should not contain a conditioner because the conditioner coats the hair and may protect the nits). It might be necessary to repeat this process after a couple of days to eliminate the next batch of hatched lice and maybe again after that. In addition to direct control of the lice on the scalp, you also need to wash clothing and linen that might be infected and dry it on high heat in a dryer. Vacuuming of carpets, sofas and chairs is regarded as an effective way of removing loose lice and nits. Combs and brushes need to be soaked in a hot ammonia solution (1 teaspoon ammonia in two cups of hot water). Head lice cannot survive for more than a couple of days at room temperature without feeding on blood, and the nits (eggs) take about 8 days to develop. Isolating items for about 10 days at warm temperatures is therefore an effective way of ridding them of any stray lice or nits. Putting an item in a plastic bag in the sun would kill lice and nits because of the high temperatures. Freezing the items for about four days would also kill the lice and nits.

Pediculus in Homeopathy

Dr. Mure introduced the remedy into homeopathy from Brazil

Rubrics with Pediculus as only remedy:
MIND; CHEERFULNESS, gaiety, happiness; tendency; afternoon; three pm. (SI-130) (1) *
MIND; DREAMS; black; forms; darkening the sun (1) *
MIND; DREAMS; body, body parts; nose; discharge, watery (SIII-282) (1) *
MIND; DREAMS; famine, being left in a dungeon to die of, escaping by crawling out (SIII-298) (hunger) (1) *
MIND; DREAMS; friendly, being (SIII-303) (1) *
MIND; DREAMS; monstrous; figure, black, that flew up to sky and darkened the sun (1) *
MIND; DREAMS; skating in the water (SIII-349) (water) (1) *
MIND; DREAMS; water; skating in summer with water up to thighs, of seeing people (1) *
MIND; DREAMS; water; wading in; acquaintances, of seeing (1) *
MIND; DREAMS; water; walking; on, acquaintances (SI-367) (1) *
MIND; HURRY, haste; tendency; writing, in; evening (1) *
MIND; STARTING, startled; evening; lying, when, and when sitting (1) *
HEAD; HAIR; affections of; horripilation, left side (1) *
HEAD; HAIR; affections of; lifted up by the hair, as if (1) *
EAR; NOISES in; whizzing; whistling, when (1) *
MOUTH; PAIN; pricking; tongue, edges (1) *
FEMALE; PAIN; General; uterus; leaning on it (1) *
FEMALE; PAIN; General; uterus; shifting (1) *
RESPIRATION; DIFFICULT; afternoon; four pm.; six pm., until (1) *
EXTREMITIES; DISCOLORATION; pale; hand; spots (1) *
EXTREMITIES; ERUPTIONS; pimples; foot; bathing in hot water (1) *
EXTREMITY PAIN; LOWER LIMBS; Knee; patella; left (1) *
SLEEP; YAWNING; afternoon; agg. three pm.; eight pm., until (SIII-218) (1) *
CHILL; COLDNESS; body, of (see SKIN; Coldness - Icy Coldness) (1) *
GENERALITIES; FAINTNESS, fainting; tendency; forenoon; nine am. (SII-180) (1) *
GENERALITIES; NUMBNESS; externally; evening (1) *
GENERALITIES; NUMBNESS; externally; inspiration, on (1) *

GENERALITIES; TREMBLING; afternoon; five pm. (SII-645) (1) *

Rubrics, that include pediculus, pulex, cimex and hirudo and thus can be considered very typical for parasites:
MIND; IRRITABILITY (K57, SI-653, G46) (Anger) (Contrary) (Contradict; disposition to) (Discontented) (Discouraged; irritability) (Quarrelsomeness) (Sensitive) (Sulky) (Unfriendly) (492)
GENERALITIES; ALTERNATING states (SII-31) (Change; symptoms) (Contradictory) (Metastasis) (44)
GENERALITIES; FOOD and drinks; meat; desires (K485, SII-255, G414) (66)

Rubrics with pediculus in third grade:
EYE; PHOTOPHOBIA; sunlight (K262, G220) (daylight) (Pain; general; light - sunlight agg.) (41) ***
EYE; PHOTOPHOBIA (K261, G220) (Pain; general; light agg.) (MIND; Light; shuns) (MIND; Sensitive; light) (218) ***

Rubrics with pediculus in second grade
MIND, AILMENTS from; joy; excessive (K60, SI-20, G48) (21) **
MIND; BOTHERSOME (7) **
MIND; DREAMS; pursued, of being (K1242, SIII-337, G1025) (fleeing) (running) (29) **
MIND; FEAR; water, of (K48, SI-532, G38) (Hydrophobia) (38) **
EXTREMITIES; ERUPTIONS; desquamation (K986, G825) (61) **
EXTREMITIES; ERUPTIONS; desquamating; foot (K1003, G837) (14) **
GENERALITIES; ALTERNATING states (SII-31) (Change; symptoms) (Contradictory) (Metastasis) (44) **
GENERALITIES; EXERTION, physical; amel. (K1358, SII-177, G1121) (Activity; amel.) (Motion; amel. rapid, running, dancing) (Running amel.) (MIND; Exertion; physical; amel.) (Walking; amel.) (40) **
GENERALITIES; FOOD and drinks; meat; desires; raw (7) **
GENERALITIES; VACCINATION; after (K1410, SII-672, G1163) (EYE; Inflammation; vaccination, after) (RECTUM; Diarrhoea; vaccination, after) (RESPIRATION; Asthmatic; vaccination, after) (EXTREMITIES; Paralysis; Lower limbs; vaccination, after) (39) **
Analysing rubrics and cases (see below) the following themes seem important
WATER

DESIRE FOR MEAT

PERSECUTION

AFFECTIONS OF HAIR

DESQUAMATING ERUPTIONS

SUNLIGHT

Case Pediculus: Child female 8 years

She is intelligent looking and a quickly reacting child. Her parents come with her. She has no intention to see a doctor. Her main complaints are alopecia and vitiligo affecting her hands mainly. She doesn't seem to care about her alopecia but she doesn't want Massimo to look at her hands. The main impression: she is very capricious, spoiled and pampered. Her parents are not able to control her. They are a nice family. "The alopecia has been present for some weeks ago. Some months ago there was a problem.

The child reacts quickly. "This is not true at all."

"There was a sunstroke after being with someone she wanted to impress. She usually always shunned the light, in this occasion she stayed outside. She hates to admit that she doesn't tolerate the sun. She is nervous in the sun. Once she even got cystitis. That day we were in the sun and she wanted to exhibit. All of a sudden she fainted when she got close to the shade. She fell into the water. She has an obsessive thought about the idea of drowning. There were nightmares and then the alopecia. We went to the psychologist, but she did not want to go. "

"I hate fish. And insects. You know "EXODUS from EGYPT", where the children were dying. I get such dreams about grasshoppers - everything becomes completely dark like before a rain and the grasshoppers might fall down"

"We worked in Africa. She must have her father kiss her otherwise her dreams come. This lasted for months. When she was younger, she suffered from a neurodermitis aggravated by sugar. The vitiligo began after cortisone treatment of ND. The vitiligo is concerning her genitals, knees, elbows and hands. Beside the allergy she has had cystitis several times since she was little.

She is very obstinate. She obtains what she wants every time. "Lawyers don't make enough money," she says. She wants to work only 6 months a years and have 6 months vacation.

There is an awful smell to the urine. She was actually quite proud of it. The itching was everywhere.

She never could endure any light, not only the sun. She has alternating states. She can be very sick, then very well. Then she will be very sick again and then very well again.

"I have been crazy for meat since I was a child. I like red and raw meat. Fruit, vegetables and milk disgust me. Only tomatoes are OK".

She did not accept any baby food. She would only eat the meat preparation for kids. She is very voracious and greedy. She has no sense of measure. She wants everything or nothing. That is true also in her mood. I think it is a mayor defect. She is hurried and stubborn. Her father is spoiling her. At school it is difficult for her to keep any friendships. She is very egoistical.

Case male, 53 years, mechanical engineer

He was very insistent on the telephone to get an appointment immediately, although his pathology was not so urgent. Massimo gave him an appointment two months later. He talks with a complaining voice. He is wearing sunglasses like Ray Charles for no apparent reason.

"I cannot wear any shoes or I am not able to walk because of my mycosis. Also I have falling of my hair. That is even more prominent than my mycosis. I have had skin troubles for a long time. It is a serious problem. Some months ago I had the fear of being poisoned. I have a hepatitis C, and had a B, too. Years ago I had a cholecystitis. I had jaundice preceded by sudden attack of itching. Even at dinner with a nice lady I had to run immediately to the toilet to scratch. There were no eruptions. As a child I had different eczemas, which went away when I stopped eating fruit. My physical efficiency is really important for my work and me. The itching concerns my hands and the back of my feet. My skin falls off (desquamation.) Between my toes, the skin is completely broken, with bleeding cracks. My feet perspire a lot and I suffer from athlete's foot. There is a strange alternation between perspiration and complete dryness. It goes - wet and dry and wet and dry. I had hepatitis and then asthmatic troubles for long time. It was a disaster. Then after an accident with my bicycle I started to stammer. That taught me to talk more calmly but now I can eat my words if I don't take care. Mostly when I am angry or excited, I stumble and stammer and I am not able to continue. I look like a stupid guy."

What about your losing hair?

"I am very irritated. For that I follow a treatment with someone else."

What does it mean to you?

"This is something really difficult. It is impossible for me to watch myself in the mirror without hair. I had a very unlucky life and now that I can start to taste my life."

What do you mean?

"Everybody is taking profit from me. (The reality is quite the contrary.) I am working like crazy and in my life I did a lot of things to reach a high position."

What do you mean?

"I don't even trust my own shadow. If I have to sign a contract, I write it myself before, because I don't want to have the risk of changing my mind in front of the person. (He is a kind of shark and has to do with poor people who would pity any other person but him. He writes the contract before so that he doesn't care whatever poor person might be in front of him.) My life was such a struggle for me; I am a very fastidious person. If I want to reach a certain goal I must arrive there. I don't surrender at all.

With women?

At this moment his face was red, tense and very irritated.

"I was married but it did not last long. My wife cost me a fortune. She said I was only thinking about money. I say she was only thinking about spending my money. For me, money is very important. I come from a humble family. I don't want to work all my life as I am doing now."

He was completely furious now. He took off his glasses and looked directly into my eyes.

"Listen to me very well. I want to solve this problem of my feet!! All the questions that you ask, I don't know where you want to arrive at, probably somewhere, but I have to do something else. So if you can do something for my hair I will be very happy."

I wanted to provoke him.

Yes, I have understood, can you say something about your relationship with light?

"Light? I cannot endure light at all. I feel well with sunglasses. I am a kind of vampire. I work in the night and sleep during the day. I am much more active during the night. Scandinavia in winter, this is my climate. Me and the sun we are not good friends, but does it make sense with my feet?"
He was very irritated.

Comments

Some of the above-mentioned symptoms are represented by the cases:
PHOTOPHOBIA
MEAT, Desire for
DESQUAMATING ERUTPIONS
AFFECTIONS OF HAIR
SUN; DARKENED NY BLACK FORMS
WATER
ALTERNATION very well/ very sick -wet/dry - work/vacation
New themes according to the cases:
A clear MATERIALISTIC ATTITUDE, greed,
EGOTISM;
Sticking to one theme, following just one idea, OBSTINACY
DICTATORIAL, not such a direct contact with others beside that he wants to take a profit of them
CAPRICIOUSNESS, I want you to do exactly what I need
Problems with the digestion of FRUIT
SKIN problems with ITCHING
LAMENTING and complaining and needing to show that he/she is sick. The purpose is to show a weak side in order to get exactly what they need/want.
Affectionate: choose to cultivate the relation with the victim. It is important for me to maintain you (the victim) in the best possible way.
He/she is less lonely than the other parasites
OFFENSIVENESS

There are 4 factors, that kill lice:
Water, sun, baldness, vinegar (which comes from fruit)
All four aspects are found to be significant in the two cases, who did very well on the homeopathic remedy "PEDICULUS HUMANUS".

PULEX IRRITANS

Traditional names:

English: Flea
German: Floh
French: puce
Dutch: vlo

Classification:

Phylum: arthropods
Class: insects-hexapods
Order: wingless insects
Family: fleas-aphaniptera

Description:

Sucking-stinging insects, hind legs are transformed into jumping legs. They lay their eggs into joins in the floor, the larvae feed on organic waste, and the adults suck blood. The flea, species pulex irritans, lives on humans, rats and poultry. It has a length of 3 mm, has a hard skin and is able to leap 35 cm in length and 20 cm in height. Fleas can fast for months. The stings cause an intense itch.

Most common species of fleas:
Men's flea -Pulex irritans
Dog's flea - Ctenocephalides canis
Cat's flea -Ctenocephalides felis
Tropical rat's flea - Xenopsylla cheopis
Poultry's flea - Ceratophyllus gallinae
Rabbit's flea -   Spilopsyllus   cuniculi
Mole's Flea - Hystrichopsylla talpae
Hedgehog's Flea - Archaeopsyllus erinacei

Geographic distribution
Worldwide, although in areas over 2000 meter sea level or in dry desert climate or conditions, where the permanent temperature stays below 4 Celsius or above 35 Celsius we will seldom meet a flea.

Host spectrum:
Humans, canids, felids, rats, pigs, hedgehogs, rodents, badgers, poultry, birds.
Adult fleas in general live exclusively as parasites of warm blooded animals, especially mammals, although birds may also be attacked. Whilst they show a certain degree of host preference, fleas are by no means specific and will feed on other animals in the absence of the normal host. In fact they tend to be more nest- than host-specific, for whilst the adults may feed on the blood of a variety of animals the larvae require more precise conditions which are associated with the habitats and nesting habits of the hosts rather than the characteristics of their blood. Cat fleas are responsible for most flea infestations, the remainder being attributable to a variety of bird and animal species. Pulex irritans infestations are now uncommon. The increased number of pets being kept and the tendency for their beds to be neglected during cleaning explain this current significance of Ctenocephalides felis. Wall-to-wall carpeting also provides a relatively undisturbed environment for flea larvae to develop, whilst the spread of central heating has served to ensure ideal temperature conditions.

Morphology
Adults – 2 - 3.25 mm long, laterally flattened, covered with backward-directed bristles, dark brown, wingless, piercing-sucking mouthparts, no combs, curved or rounded head, with long, powerful back legs fitted with very large coxae, 5-jointed tarsi, and large claws. The human flea lacks the genal and pronotal combs characteristic of the cat flea and dog flea, and may be distinguished from the oriental rat flea by having its ocular bristle inserted beneath the eye instead of in front of it, as it is in the latter species.

Life cycle (stages)
Eggs, larvae, pupae:
A female flea will lay 4 to 8 eggs after each blood meal, and can usually lay several hundred eggs during her adult life. The smooth, oval or rounded, light-collared eggs, about 0.5 mm long, are deposited on, but not firmly attached to, the body, the bedding, or the nest of the host. Although they are a little sticky,

those laid on the host's body may fall or be brushed off. This accounts for their being found in crevices in the floor, under the edges of carpeting, in sofas, or in cat or dog boxes, kennels, etc., where they usually hatch in 10 days or less.

The small, hairy, wormlike larvae, are whitish, with a distinct, brownish head, and do not have eyes or legs. They have 3 thoracic and 10 abdominal segments, with a single row of bristles around each segment. The larvae are about 1.5 mm long when they emerge, finally becoming about 5 mm long. They move forward by using their backward-projecting bristles and a pair of hooked, chitinous processes located at the end of the abdomen by which they can obtain purchase on a surface. When disturbed, they may "flip" in circles to escape. The larvae of some species require dried blood for food, but others do not. Those that do not need blood can feed on the many kinds of organic debris that are present in the crevices in which the eggs commonly hatch. They also feed on their own cast skins. They require high humidity. Within a week to several months, the larvae grow through 3 instars, and then spin a pupal cocoon covered with grains of sand, dust, or organic debris, in which they are quite effectively camouflaged in their natural surroundings.

The pupae are initially white, but they change to brownish before the adults emerge. In the pupa, the appendages are not closely pressed to the body, and it has the general shape and characteristics of the adult. Under favourable conditions, the adult emerges in a week or two, but under adverse conditions, the pupal period may be prolonged to as much as a year. The adult may remain in the cocoon for a long time until vibrations indicating the presence of a possible host stimulate it to emerge and become active. Adult fleas are also able to detect the body heat of a new host by a heat-sensing organ on their posterior called the sensillum.

The potentially long pupal stage, besides the fact that adult fleas can live without food for remarkably long periods, accounts for the fact that people may enter a house after it has been unoccupied by humans or pets for months, yet be rapidly and severely attacked by fleas. Depending on the species and weather conditions, 2 or 3 weeks to as many months, and rarely as long as 2 years, are required for many species of fleas to complete a life cycle. The human flea is usually the most important species in farm areas. While the bites of the cat flea tend to be concentrated on the lower parts of the legs, those of the human flea may be generally distributed over the body (Keh and Barnes, 1961).

Other Features of the flea:

The body of the adult flea is ideally suited for gliding through the narrow spaces between the hairs of its host, being oval and greatly compressed laterally, and since the body-covering is also smooth and firm it escapes easily when an attempt is made to catch it either between the fingers of man or between the teeth of lower mammals. Once out of the clutch of an enemy, the flea quickly leaps away. It is this unusual power of leaping that enables it to transfer readily from mammal to mammal. The human flea has been known to leap for a distance of thirteen inches, and to a height of seven and three-quarter inches. An equivalent leap for a man would carry him 275 feet up into the air and 450 feet horizontally! (Extract from Reference Works: Natural History)

Site of infestation and pathogenesis/clinical signs

The bite of the flea causes irritation, scratching and restlessness. Some people react severely to fleabites, while others hardly notice them. Fleas most often bite people about the legs and ankles, and there are usually 2 or 3 bites in a row. The bites are felt immediately, but tend to become increasingly irritating, and are frequently sore for as much as a week. Fleabites may vary in their effects, from a transient wheal to prolonged symptoms that last for years, depending on the sensitivity of the victim. Children less than 10 years old were found to be more sensitive to the bites than older persons (Hudson et al., 1960b). The insects inject hemorrhagic saliva that can cause severe itching, and repeated bites may produce a generalized rash. A small, red spot usually appears where the flea's mandibles have penetrated the skin. The spot is surrounded by a red halo, but there is never much swelling. Some relief from the itching can be obtained by applying cooling preparations, such as carbolated vaseline, menthol, camphor, or calamine solution, or by placing a piece of ice on the affected area. For people who suffer severe allergic reactions, antigens are available that are sufficiently effective to cause the immunized person to be subsequently unaware of fleabites.

Disease Transmission:

The most serious indictment against fleas is their ability to transmit disease organisms. This ability is enhanced by their promiscuous feeding habits; they move from one host species to another. For example, the cat flea, Cteno-cephalides felis, readily attacks humans, dogs, rats, opossums, raccoons, and foxes. The human flea, Pulex irritans, can be found on dogs, rats, pigs, mice, skunks, badgers, deer, foxes, coyotes, prairie dogs, ground squirrels, and bur-rowing owls. The species normally found on rats and ground squirrels also bite man.

Plague:
Probably the most dreadful calamity in all human history was the "Black Death," a series of plagues of the Middle Ages, particularly in the fourteenth century. Although not known at the time, the highly contagious disease was caused by a bacillus, Yersinia pestis (= Pasteurella), carried primarily by rats and transmitted by the fleas they harboured. The disease caused swellings of the lymph glands and subcutaneous haemorrhages that turned black. The plague first struck in Asia, and then spread to Russia, Persia, Turkey, North Africa, and Europe. The Encyclopedia Britannica estimates that one-third of the world's people perished. The most dangerous forms of plague are bubonic, septicaemia, and pneumonic. Two types are named for the parts of the body infected. Bu-bonic plague, confined initially to lymphatic glands (buboes), is not so danger-ous as the septicaemia, and especially the pneumonic, phases, which are rapidly spread from person to person by airborne infection (Dubos and Hirsch, 1965). Bubonic plague is no longer a major scourge of mankind, but only because we now know how it is transmitted, and therefore how to prevent it. War and dislo-cation can still increase its potential, but not as in past centuries. The World Health Organization reported 1318 cases of plague in 1968 and 864 in 1969, the majority from Vietnam; Treatment of the disease is quite effective with modern antibiotics. However, it can sometimes be dangerous, even with early diagnosis and treatment.

The oriental rat flea, Xenopsylla cheopis, is the most important vector of the plague bacillus, Yersinia pestis, from rat to man but at least 29 other species of fleas can transit the disease including the northern rat flea, Nosopsyllus fascia-tus; the mouse flea, Leptopsylla segnis; the dog flea, Ctenocephalides canis; the cat flea, C. felis; and the human flea, Pulex irritans. Plague is transmitted while the infected flea is feeding, by regurgitation of the bacillus from the flea's ali-mentary tract through the proboscis into the new host. Yersinia pestis is rapidly eliminated from the proventriculus of the oriental rat flea when the mean monthly ambient temperature exceeds 28 °C (82 °F), and plague epidemics decline with the advent of hot weather (Cavanaugh, 1971).

"Sylvatic" or "endemic" is the designation used for the plague in wild rodents. Under certain ecological conditions in vacated squirrel burrows, fleas may continue to harbour the plague bacilli for many months, providing a reservoir for the infection. Fleas are particularly suitable for this purpose because of their remarkable longevity, for they can survive more than 6 months, even without food. Sylvatic plague occurs in many parts of the world, remaining somewhat localized in each area. A group of rodents maintains the infection, and if domiciliary rats or mice come in contact with such a focus of infection, the disease may be carried to human habitations and human cases may result. Likewise, if humans enter sylvatic plague territory, they may become infected.

Murine Typhus:
The oriental rat flea is also the principal vector of murine or endemic typhus that may be transmitted from rats to man. This disease is caused by the microorganism Rickettsia mooseri, and is widespread in rats and other rodents. The principal mode of transmission is believed to be by rubbing or scratching infected flea faeces into wounds made by their bites. Murine typhus should not be confused with the more serious epidemic typhus, which has caused the deaths of millions of persons, but is transmitted by lice. The fatality rate for murine typhus, on the other hand, is only about 2 %.
Also, new broad-spectrum antibiotics have been successful in the treatment of clinical cases of the disease (Pratt and Wiseman, 1962).

Tapeworms:
Fleas, particularly dog and cat fleas, can serve as intermediate hosts for the dog tapeworm, Dipylidium caninum (L.), and the rodent tapeworm, Hymenolepis diminuta (Rudolphi), which occasionally attack humans, particularly very young children.

History, legends, traditional use:

The name Pulex was given to the human flea by the Romans because of their mistaken belief that fleas originated from pulvis, or dirt. Also Aristotle's and the middle age were convinced that the flea directly came from dirt. The traditional name flea, German "Floh" is related to the verb to flee, in german "fliehen". Another old word for flea is in old English "loppa" Swedish "loppa", Danish "loppe" which means "the runner, the jumper". The roman names such as French "puce", Italian "pulce", Spanish "pulga" all originate from the Latin name pulex.

Fleas have been a plague for mankind for thousands of years. The living conditions of our ancestors, especially of those who lived in a primitive way, have favoured the offensive presence of the flea. The flea has always been the embodiment of quickness, importunity, inconvenience and smallness. In nearly all languages there exists a special expression for flea hunting, e.g. old German: "vloehenen" italien "spulgiare" etc. Believing that the flea originated from dirt, Beelzebub, god of the dirt, was the master of the vermin. In the language of the soldiers the flea was called black dragonet, black rider, or brown dragoon, referring to the colour of the animal. On the other hand the name was used to describe certain persons. In the language of the Parisian argot "puce" was the name for a Spanish or a black woman. The Spanish called a nervous person "pülguilla", whereas the Italian know the expression "occhi di pulce".

The name of several plants remind of the flea, such as Flohalant (Inula pulicaria), Flohhaber (Avena sterilis), Flohknöterich (Polygonum amphibium), Flohkraut (Mentha pulegium), Flohpfeffer (Polygonum hydropiper), Flohsame (Plantago psyllion). Probably some of them were used to relieve the ailments caused by the fleas.

Flea circus:
Fleas seem to be quite intelligent and can be trained by a certain procedure. Their great strength in relation to their size allows fleas to pull miniature carts and perform other stunts in 'flea circuses' - popular in Victorian times but still performed by some entertainers. In reward for their work they may suck blood from their owner.

Homeopathy:

Used parts: the whole animal

Themes of pulex:

Egotism, selfishness, idea of profit.

NEED FOR CHANGE; RESTLESSNESS
Greediness
Disgust, dissatisfaction
Aversion to company

Swelling, swelling personalities
Chilliness
OFFENSIVENESS OF SECRETIONS AND BODYFLUIDS

Old appearance
Craving for meat, desire for icy drinks
Burning and stitching pains:
Symptoms in the urogenitaltract
ENLARGEMENT OF THE EYES

Egotism, selfishness, idea of profit

As in all the other bloodsuckers the tendency of selfishness is strongly represented in pulex. Using other people for their purposes without any scruples is typical for patients who need this remedy. They are not interested in feelings such as love or sympathy. What really counts is their personal profit; they are cold and selfish persons.

NEED FOR CHANGE, RESTLESSNESS

What is typical for pulex is the need to change the environment or the life style very often. It could be a constant change of partners or professions; it could also be the need to move from one town to the other. In any case there is a strong desire to taste everything in life, remaining always unsatisfied, so they have to go further. Pulex patients are "jumping" personalities, (once again the similarity to the behaviour of the animal is seen in the remedy) personalities who never have enough. This could be underlined by the sentence of a patient, an actress, who said: " You need to go so deeply into your role that you even are able to taste what the person tastes. You have to enter so much into this personality to know what is really going on.

So you may jump from one personality to another. Another expression of the restlessness is the impatience of pulex. They have to get what they want immediately, waiting makes them even more cross than they are already. A certain haughtiness, which lays in their behaviour, could also increase their impatience towards others, expecting the others to react according to their wishes.

But it is not only impatience towards the others but towards life itself.

MIND; ADULT
MIND; HAUGHTY
MIND; IRRITABILITY
MIND; MOROSE,
MIND; IMPATIENCE
GENERALITIES; ALTERNATING states

Disgust, dissatisfaction

Although or precisely because they try to taste everything from life by jumping from one situation or person to the other they remain unsatisfied. A feeling of loneliness, inner coldness and disgust easily takes possession of them. This feeling of disgust is not only expressed on a mental level but also physically. We find it in symptoms as offensive leucorrhoea, offensive perspiration, offensive urine, which is experienced as disgusting, also disgusting taste of saliva, as described in both cases. Not only the secretions of the body are offensive but as well the behaviour of pulex may be in some way offensive and penetrating. These patients do not accept social limits, they are complaining easily, they are intrusive and demanding, it is not so easy to get rid of them. Once again the nature of the flea, being so intrusive in getting its food as well as the fact that it comes out of the dirt and transmits diseases which makes the animal disgusting, is very near. Perhaps it is due to these feelings of disgust and dissatisfaction, which lead to the old-looking expression in the face of pulex. It is typical to look older and often they feel older then they are.

STOOL; ODOR; offensive
URINE; ODOR; offensive
FEMALE; LEUCORRHEA; offensive
PERSPIRATION; ODOR; offensive
TASTE; METALLIC
FACE; EXPRESSION; old looking

Greediness

Greediness, a common theme of all the bloodsuckers, is expressed in pulex by this way of jumping from one subject, experience or person to the other to take what they need. They want to live everything, which is possible in life, but remain unsatisfied. Greediness is characterized by the feeling of never getting enough. Even when they are full they already feel an emerging emptiness or a kind of dissatisfaction. In some way they are always hungry, and try to tease their hunger by experiences, in which they are the taking part. Hirudo tries to tease hunger by eating always more than needed, or by filling himself up with material goods.

Aversion to company

Usually they do not lead deeper relationships They rather prefer to change their partners very often, after having taken from them what they wanted to have, after having sucked them out. They are not interested in deeper contact; in these relationships each one remains lonely. The idea of a bloodsucker, which takes from its victim without regard, is mostly evident. Pulex is not interested in destroying the other person. Possessing a kind of "Dracula" mentality, pulex needs his victim alive.

Swelling, swelling personalities

Pulex belongs to the class of the insects. Which have symptoms as swelling, burning, itching and restlessness in common. On a physical level the enlargement of the eyes, or the feeling as if the eyes could come out because of being so big and swollen, seems to be characteristic. After the sting of insects intense swelling often occurs. On a mental level they show themselves as swelling characters, with all their haughtiness and demanding, offensive attitude. They have to fill up their emptiness inside by "swelling" in front of the others.

MIND; HAUGHTY

EYE; ENLARGEMENT, sensation of

SKIN; STINGS of insects

Chilliness

"Coldness is an inner dimension", said a patient who needed pulex. The physical chilliness is strongly related to an emotional coldness, a coldness that is felt inside. It cannot be relieved from outside. In a warm environment the perception of the inner coldness is even increased, which is expressed by rubrics as " chill, besides fire agg". Or "chilliness from heat of stove". Even the rubrics "flushes of heat, as if being over steam" and "pain burning externally like over steam" could be interpreted in that sense: The difference between the inner coldness and the warmer environment is so enormous, that the temperature outside is perceived as hot as steam, which may cause a burning pain externally.

CHILL; CHILLINESS
CHILL; CHILLINESS; stove, heat of, from
CHILL; FIRE, besides, agg.
CHILL; WARMTH; desire for, which does not relieve
GENERALITIES; HEAT; flushes of; steam, being over as if
GENERALITIES; PAIN; burning; externally; steam, over, like

Offensiveness of secretions and body fluids

Characteristic is the offensiveness of all secretions and body fluids. The odour is penetrating and evokes disgust, not only in other people but also in the person himself. The discharge may even stain the linen as mentioned in relation with leucorrhoea. It may be burning, like acid. As the theme of disgust, penetration and offensiveness is really fundamental in pulex it is expressed everywhere in the body. It may concern stool, urine, leucorrhoea or sweat. Even the taste of saliva is disgusting, often combined with increased salivation and a strong desire to spit.

TASTE; METALLIC
STOOL; ODOR; offensive
STOOL; ODOR; putrid
URINE; ODOR; offensive
FEMALE; LEUCORRHEA; offensive
FEMALE; LEUCORRHEA; purulent
FEMALE; LEUCORRHEA; staining the linen

FEMALE; MENSES; wash off, difficult to
PERSPIRATION; ODOR; offensive
GENERALITIES; DISCHARGES, secretions; stain indelibly fast
MOUTH; SALIVATION

Old appearance

Even young people look older than they are. It is certainly due to the inner experience of feeling old that makes the face wrinkled and old looking.

FACE; EXPRESSION; old looking
FACE; WRINKLED

Craving for meat, desire for icy drinks

As in all the other bloodsuckers we find a craving for meat, sometimes even raw meat and a strong desire for icy cold drinks, which ameliorate. Both symptoms are not expressed in the repertory but descend from clinical experience.

Burning and stitching pains:

As already mentioned above, the character of the symptoms is mostly burning, itching, stitching and swelling, as we know it from the insects.

FEMALE; PAIN; burning
FEMALE; PAIN; burning; vagina
SKIN; ITCHING
GENERALITIES; PAIN; burning; externally
GENERALITIES; PAIN; burning; externally; steam, over, like
GENERALITIES; PAIN; stitching

Symptoms in the urogenitaltract

Physically the symptoms are concentrated on the urogenitaltract, reminding us that pulex belongs to the class of the insects. So it is not surprising that there is a remarkably high amount of rubrics in the repertory concerning the urogenital tract in comparison with the number of rubrics in general. All in all 67 rubrics are described, 15 rubrics we find in the female genital tract, and 11 rubrics concern bladder and urine.

<u>Bladder, urethra</u>:

Burning, swelling and stitching pains with an urging desire to urinate are described. The odour of the urine is offensive as all the secretions of pulex. Ailments of the bladder may occur before and during menses.

BLADDER; IRRITABILITY
BLADDER; IRRITABILITY; menses, before
BLADDER; MENSES, ailments before and during
BLADDER; PAIN; General
BLADDER; PAIN; pressing, pressure in
BLADDER; URGING to urinate, morbid desire
BLADDER; URGING to urinate, morbid desire; frequent
BLADDER; URINATION; interrupted, intermittent
BLADDER; URINATION; interrupted, intermittent; suddenly, then followed
by pain
BLADDER; WEAKNESS
URINE; ODOR; offensive
URINE; SCANTY

<u>Female genital tract</u>:

Genital infections with profuse, offensive discharge and burning pains seem to be one of the most important symptoms on a physical level. It is frequently mentioned that the leucorrhoea is not only offensive but also stains the linen.

FEMALE; BALL; vagina, in, like cotton
FEMALE; LEUCORRHEA; General
FEMALE; LEUCORRHEA; greenish
FEMALE; LEUCORRHEA; offensive
FEMALE; LEUCORRHEA; profuse
FEMALE; LEUCORRHEA; purulent
FEMALE; LEUCORRHEA; staining the linen
FEMALE; LEUCORRHEA; staining the linen; indelibly
FEMALE; LEUCORRHEA; yellow
FEMALE; LEUCORRHEA; yellow; stains linen
FEMALE; MENSES; green

FEMALE; MENSES; late, too
FEMALE; MENSES; wash off, difficult to
FEMALE; PAIN; burning
FEMALE; PAIN; burning; vagina

SENSATION OF ENLARGEMENT OF THE EYES

The sensation of enlargement of the eyes, which seem to come out, is typical in pulex.

Sometimes it may be related to a headache.

EYE; ENLARGEMENT, sensation of

First case: A young woman, 21 years old

Appearance seductive, rough and rude. In the waiting room she was complaining at the secretary, because she wanted to be treated immediately. A very friendly woman accompanied her. She looks older than her age and her way of speaking is like this of a business lady of 40 years. She said that she got the telephone number from her gynaecologist.

"It is a recurrent thing. I want to make it clear; I have not so much patience. Several years ago it started. I have had a leucorrhoea all the time. Trichomonades, candida and streptococci were found. With a diet (no milk, no coffee etc) it was better, but they did not take away my beloved meat, unless I would not have done it. During the diet meat felt like a stone in the stomach and afterwards I got a headache. Sometimes I had to vomit to wash the stone out of my stomach. I always drink something very cold which helps me to digest and I often have to spit because the taste in my mouth is so awful. Now after the diet I still have a headache and the infection came back again. When I have the infection I cannot work. I hate when I am not able to work, because I want to work. I am a gym-teacher just for women and I cannot jump when I have the infection because it hurts in my ovaries when I am jumping. Now I have to deal with fat old women and look after the machines. I am the owner of the gym studio; my father bought it for me. I have such a burning pain in my urethra. I have to run to urinate, unless it is too late. It is a crazy burning and there is this awful smell of my urine too. My stool also has an awful smell. The burning is so strong that I cannot keep the urine inside. I tried to keep it but then it is even worse. The urine is like acid, and I often have a strong burning between the labiae and in the whole vagina too. Leucorrhoea with bad smell is humiliating. "

During the consultation she always tries to change topic and wants to direct the conversation.

"I am homosexual, I do not regard men so highly, but in general I do not highly regard human beings. I am a person, who has thousands of passions, when I have the desire to do something I do it. When I enjoyed it thoroughly I have to do something new. I would like to leave the gym studio but I got sick, probably because I do not want to loose my face. All these complaints show me that I am not well. I am a chronically dissatisfied person. I always had an awful relationship with my father. He is very rich. He always wanted to work with me but then I had a love affair with the secretary of my father and I made him pay me money not to tell anybody that I am lesbian. My father had already chosen a husband for me, who was very rich too. I made my parents crazy. I changed school six times, afterwards I began to study medicine, and then biology and afterwards I became a gym-teacher. I had a relationship with a married man, a business partner of my father, before I became lesbian. One experience is not enough for me. Even one life is not enough. I never was able to do something that really satisfied me. I do one thing until the end and then I have to change and find something new. Each time I think this time I will start completely new and will do it in a different way but then it is always the same. I feel very old inside. Probably in the future I could be committed to another person. In some way a real relationship is a kind of social dying for me. I feel my solitude a lot, but more than my solitude I feel the solitude of the people who are attracted by me. I attract only very lonely people. I do not change at all. I become so stubborn, until I get what I want. I want to do something great but I do not want to become a fossil and always do the same. I am not stupid. I know when I have to go. There are enough stupid nuns and priests on this planet who love to suffer, me not.

If a headache does not stop I even would take morphine to get rid of my pains. If I have my menses I always take painkillers .To make my headache better I drink wine and then I go to bed. I often have a dream when I have my headache that my eyes are coming out of my head and I look like a frog -it is horrible. Frogs are my favourite animals. They are swelling in front of their enemies and make them stupid. They do not run, not walk but just jump. Jumping is a good way of moving. Nevertheless frogs do not jump far enough, this does not satisfy me. I am extremely chilly, esp. when I go to sleep. Coldness is an inner dimension. I become so nervous because nothing can heat me.

Second case: an actress, 44 years old

Beautiful appearance, rough and haughty behaviour. She wants to be treated immediately; she does not want to be recognized.

"For a long time I have gynaecological problems. Now I have an awful leucorrhoea and I do not want to take "poisons": I have a terrible burning and itching. If I follow my personal diet it is better, I have my own diet to keep my weight. I cannot endure that I am destroying my precious underwear. There must be acid in my blood. It started after a bladder infection, which was treated with antibiotics because I had to work. Afterwards I also had diarrhoea with vomiting and itching. The only thing I can do for my digestion is to drink a glass of icy cold water or a glass of wine. Afterwards I sleep, and then it is okay. I love meat, I am a meat-eater. When the leucorrhoea starts I often have a disgusting taste in my mouth. My urine still has a very bad smell. For 3 days I had such a pain in my head as if my eyes would jump out. I often have this headache with pain in my eyes.

Usually I am a very overactive person but now I have no ambition to work. I would like to stay in bed all the time. I have a kind of allergy; there is such an enormous swelling after a mosquito bite. Sleep is fine. I have had a dream since I was a child: I jumped from one house to the other, when my parents were quarrelling. I grew up in a horrible family; there were a lot of quarrels. This was no problem for me, but rather the possibility to get everything I wanted twice. My parents were dependent on me. There I started to be an actress. I am a cold and cynical person. That is what I heard from all my lovers. I just think of my career. Is it wrong? My ideal is Robert de Niro. You need to go so deeply into your role that you even are able to taste what the person tastes. You have to enter so much into this personality to know what is really going on. So you may jump from one personality to another. That is what I always wanted since I was a child.

HIRUDO MEDICINALIS

Traditional names:
English: medicinal leech
German: Blutegel

Classification:

Kingdom: animalia
Phylum: annelida
Class: oligochaeta
Order: gnathobdellida
Family: Hirudinidae
Genus: hirudo
Species: hirudo medicinalis

Description:

The leech is a blood sucking annelid worm, reaching a length of 20 cm. It may achieve an age of 20 years, if kept under good conditions. It has a cylindrical, dorsoventrally flattened body divided into thirty-three or thirty-four segments. The dorsal side is dark brown or black, bearing six longitudinal, reddish or brown stripes, and the ventral surface is speckled. All members bear a posterior and anterior disk-shaped sucker. The anterior sucker surrounds the oral opening where the teeth for incision are located. In addition, the medicinal leech has five pairs of testes and one pair of ovaries as well as a thickening of the body ring, known as a clitellum, which is visible during the breeding season.

Geographic range:
The range extends through parts of western and southern Europe to the Ural Mountains and the countries bordering the northeastern Mediterranean. The medicinal leech is rare throughout its range in Europe and extinct in much of its former range. This is due primarily to the over harvesting of leeches in the past century for medicinal use. Other factors contributing to the leech's reduced

status is the alteration of its usual habitat and possibly a decrease in the frog population.

Habitat:

The medicinal leech is amphibious, needing both land and water, and resides exclusively in fresh water. A typical habitat for H. medicinalis would be a small pond with a muddy bottom edged with reeds and in which frogs are at least seasonally abundant.

Food habits:

The leech is parasitic and the adults feed on the blood of mammals. It attaches to the host by means of its two suckers and bites through the skin of its victim. Simultaneously, the leech injects an anaesthetic so that its presence is not detected, and an anticoagulant in order for the incision to remain open during the meal. It has three jaws, which work back and forth during the feeding process, which usually lasts about 20 to 40 minutes and leaves a tripartite star-shaped scar on the host. After a full meal of 10 ml to 15 ml of blood, the medicinal leech may increase 5 to 8 times its initial body size. After a meal it may occur that the leech vomits a part of the blood. H.medicinalis often attacks the orifices of the victims body - nose, mouth, even throat and sinuses. Leeches only feed about once every six months, this is about how long the blood meal takes to be fully digested. Certain bacteria, esp. pseudomonahirudinis, keep the blood from decaying during the long digestion period. H. medicinalis may even go up to 2 years without food by digesting its own tissues. Young leeches feed on cold-blooded animals, such as fish and frogs instead of mammals because their jaws are not yet strong enough to cut through mammalian skin.

Reproduction:

Leeches are hermaphrodites. Each individual produces both eggs and sperm. This does not happen simultaneously, so that self-fertilization does not occur. A leech first functions as a male and then as a female. H. medicinalis breeds once during an annual season that spans June through August. It also remains fertile over the period of years, unlike most other leech species. The act of copulation takes place on land, where one leech attaches ventrally to one another by means of a mucus secretion. Sperm is injected into the vagina by an extendable copulatory organ. A cocoon is formed around the clitellum and slips off the anterior section of the leech. The whole egg sac is laid in damp soil usually just above the shoreline. After about 14 days, the eggs hatch as fully formed miniature adults.

Behaviour:
Motility is achieved both in land and water. H. medicinalis moves in water by contraction of the longitudinal muscles of the body in a wave-like motion which propels it forward in the water. Movement on land is accomplished by means of "looping", a movement similar to that of inchworms. They attach themselves to the substrate alternately by their anterior and posterior suckers. While at rest, the medicinal leech lies under large objects on the shoreline, partially out of water. The leech is able to detect the movement of shadows above. Especially when hungry it will respond to moving shadows, which often indicate a source of mammalian food. The leech is sensitive to light, heat, dryness and dissection. It becomes desensitised during feeding and copulation to the point where the posterior end can be cut off and it will continue the same behaviour. Nevertheless mostly you can force a leech to detach from a body by holding a lighted match or a burning cigarette to its body or by putting some salt on it. In daylight they can adapt their colour to the surroundings.

Toxicology, pharmacy, medicine

The medicinal leech, as its name suggests, has historically been used for medical purposes, mainly to remove "bad blood" from the diseased. The saliva of the leech contains hirudin and heparin, which inhibits blood coagulation. The bite is anaesthetizing and induces the reconstruction of capillaries. Usually it is, in contrary to other bloodsucking animal, a "healthy" bite without transmission of diseases. Nevertheless a transmission of diseases by the bite cannot be excluded completely if the leech was fed with contaminated blood before. When a leech sucks, the blood mixes up with the saliva of the leech Therefore serious bleeding may occur after the bite of a leech. Medically it has always been used for purposes of induced bleeding and dilution. In the past every physician carried with him a lancet and a leech. Around 1850 this practice fell into disrepute, but H.medicinalis has again become of value in medicinal practices. It is used now for the treatment and prophylaxis of thrombosis and emboli, inflammatory processes, rheumatic diseases, angina pectoris and migraine. The anticoagulant of leeches is also a fertile ground of research for surgeries in which an incision must be kept open. In addition leech saliva is found to contain powerful antibiotics and anaesthetics which no doubt will prove useful in future medicinal practice.

Homeopathy:

Original proving:

Done by Raeside in 1961 with 18 people, 9 men and 9 women, afterwards by Sankaran with 12 persons
Used parts:
The end of the leech's head is macerated for 20 minutes in a mixture of sand and a physiological serum. Centrifuge the liquid and a green liquid residue is obtained, which is dried after addition of thymol.

Themes of hirudo:

IDEA OF GROWING, SWELLING, BURSTING
Greediness
Egotism, profit
Aversion company

Competition
Persecution
HEMORRHAGIC TENDENCY
Chilliness
Photophobia
Ravenous appetite, craving for meat

Aversion fruits, vegetables, craving for icy cold water
Cardiac diseases
gastrointestinal symptoms
symptoms in the female genital tract
headache

IDEA OF GROWING, SWELLING, BURSTING

The idea of growing, swelling and bursting is a fundamental theme of Hirudo. It is as well found on a mental as on a physical level. They are swelling and competitive personalities, in the sense of having to fill them up as much as possible. These patients often eat much more than needed, with the idea of having to grow. They never get enough. They are anxious to loose their energy if they do not get enough food and hence grow enough like the leech which sucks until it is 5 times its body weight, now able to endure the fasting period. This greedy, swelling and growing aspect is also expressed by the impulse to collect material things, to earn as much money as possible. They have no idea of measure, it is always too much, and they collect and eat until they could burst. On a physical level they may have bursting, throbbing pains, as if something could explode because of its fullness as described in the 2nd case. We also find a congestion of blood.

MIND; EATING; amel. mental symptoms
STOMACH; APPETITE; increased, hunger in general
STOMACH; APPETITE; ravenous, canine, excessive
GENERALITIES; CONGESTION of blood
HEAD; PULSATING, beating, throbbing
HEAD; PULSATING, beating, throbbing; Forehead

Greediness

The idea of greediness is strongly related with the idea of growing and the fear of loosing energy. On a physical level the loss of energy may be expressed by the strong bleeding tendency of hirudo. Loosing blood is loosing the liquid of life, or even life itself. Gaining as much blood as possible means to grow and hence to be able to survive for a longer period. The "bloodsucker-mentality", which makes us think of Dracula, or a vampire, is very characteristic for hirudo. To be able to grow as much as possible they need to be greedy to get enough. Nevertheless what they get is never enough, they do not have a feeling for the right measure. This feeling of never having enough, this lack of satisfaction makes them cross and discontent. Hirudo patients are mainly concerned by materialistic matters. They try to gain as much possession as possible. To earn a lot of money is much more attractive to them than to achieve knock ledge. Usually they are not interested in arts, they have no ambition to study or to widen their intellectual horizon otherwise. A kind of "mental possession" is not important for them.

MIND; BOTHERSOME
MIND; GREED, cupidity
MIND; GREED, cupidity; eating, in
MIND; HARSHNESS, rough
MIND; QUARRELSOMENESS, scolding
STOMACH; APPETITE; increased, hunger in general
STOMACH; APPETITE; ravenous, canine, excessive

Egotism, profit

The way to achieve their goals is a very egotistic one. Hirudopatients are lonely fighters; they avoid working in teams. Sympathy, solidarity or love does not mark out hirudo patients. It is considerable that one of the organs mostly affected is the heart, which is said to be the place of love. They do not like to share something with other people. They try to take as much as possible from them. If they see a possibility to take profit of a situation or a person they will do it even if it is to the prejudice of somebody else." To survive I just have to consider myself and nothing else and I take everything I can get from the others" - idea of vampires, of Dracula, of bloodsucking animals, which are just able to survive at the expense of somebody else. Nevertheless they are interested in their victims staying alive unless they would loose their own source of life.

MIND; SELFISHNESS, egoism

Aversion company

People who need hirudo do not like company. They are not able to lead deeper relationships. Usually they prefer to stay alone. Other people are not considered as enrichment for life but rather as an obstacle on their way to get as much profit as possible. Being cold and hard they are just interested in their own affairs. Children have no desire to play with other children. They are no team workers, co workers rather disturb them, they want to do everything for themselves sharing, friendship, love, solidarity, communication is not at all important for them. In contact with others they are quarrelsome, discontent and cross.

MIND; BOTHERSOME
MIND; GREED, cupidity

MIND; HARSHNESS, rough
MIND; QUARRELSOMENESS,
MIND; SELFISHNESS,

Competition

Competition is a consequence of the greediness. To get as much as possible they have to fight against everybody who interferes with their interests. Fairness does not belong to one of their typical qualities. To reach their aims they do not care if it is at the expense of somebody else. They may take advantage of somebody else without any scruple. Often they have high expectations towards themselves. The expectations concern mostly their ability of earning money and becoming rich. If they do not succeed they get very cross with themselves and their surrounding too.

MIND; AMBITION; much, ambitious

Persecution

There also seems to be the tendency of feeling persecuted, which is mainly represented in the dreams .In one dream the patient has to flee from a truck with burning material loaded but in front of him lies the desert and he knows that he cannot go there because the desert would kill him. Heat and fire - both elements which hirudo does not like at all.

MIND; DREAMS; pursued, of being

HEMORRHAGIC TENDENCY, DISTURBANCE OF BLOOD COAGULATION

The blood coagulation is disturbed in the sense of a strong bleeding tendency but also in the sense of increased blood clotting with thrombosis and thrombophlebitis. Concerning the haemorrhagic tendency hirudo is an important remedy for wounds, which are bleeding freely, for nose bleeding and all kinds of haemophilia. On the other hand we find thrombosis and thrombophlebitis esp. of the lower limbs. The pains are bursting and swelling. A patient with phlebitis of the lower limbs had the impression of having the leg of a hippotamus and wanted to make it bleed as most as possible.

NOSE; EPISTAXIS
GENERALITIES; HEMORRHAGE; tendency or actual
GENERALITIES; HEMORRHAGE; tendency or actual; blood; coagulate, does not, haemophilia
GENERALITIES; HEMORRHAGE; tendency or actual; blood; watery
GENERALITIES; HEMORRHAGE; tendency or actual; heart symptoms, with
GENERALITIES; HEMORRHAGE; tendency or actual; small wounds bleed much
GENERALITIES; WOUNDS; bleeding; freely
EXTREMITIES; INFLAMMATION; Veins
EXTREMITIES; INFLAMMATION; Veins; chronic
EXTREMITIES; MILK LEG, phlegmasia alba dolmens, phlebitis
EXTREMITIES; THROMBOSIS, Lower limbs
GENERALITIES; INFLAMMATION; blood vessels; phlebitis, milk leg

Chilliness

Hirudopatients are very chilly. They often feel the cold inside themselves. Their emotional frigidity seems to be perceived as a physical chilliness.

GENERALITIES; HEAT; vital, lack of

Photophobia

Photophobia is another characteristic symptom of hirudo we find an aversion against sunlight, hirudo patients prefer to stay in rooms with dim light. Further there might be an aggravation from sunlight.

EYE; PHOTOPHOBIA
EYE; PHOTOPHOBIA; sunlight
GENERALITIES; SUN, from; exposure to; agg. or ailments from

Ravenous appetite, craving for meat, esp. raw meat

Their impulse to fill themselves up, to grow and to swell becomes more than all evident in the strong appetite.

The appetite is increased, often enormous. Hirudo patients always eat more than they need. The craving for meat, esp. for raw meat, is not astonishing thinking of hirudo as a bloodsucking animal.

MIND; EATING; amel. mental symptoms
MIND; GREED, cupidity; eating, in
STOMACH; APPETITE; increased, hunger in general
STOMACH; APPETITE; ravenous, canine, excessive
GENERALITIES; FOOD and drinks; meat; desires
GENERALITIES; FOOD and drinks; meat; desires; raw

Aversion vegetables, fruits, craving for icy water

We find a strong craving for cold, icy water.
Further they dislike vegetables and fruits. Sometimes a fructose allergy may be found.

GENERALITIES; FOOD and drinks; cold; drinks, water; desires
GENERALITIES; FOOD and drinks; fruit; agg. *

Cardiac diseases, esp. after tonsillitis

A strong tendency towards heart inflammation, esp. a rheumatic endocarditis after tonsillitis is found. It might be related with a bleeding tendency. Mentionable is also aneurysm of the aorta. In general hirudo has a remarkable affinity towards the circulation system. It may be expressed as thrombosis, thrombophlebitis, inflammation of blood vessels and heart, milk leg, aneurysm or the distinct hemorrhagic tendency.

CHEST; ANEURISM of the; aorta
CHEST; INFLAMMATION; Heart
CHEST; INFLAMMATION; Heart; endocardium
CHEST; INFLAMMATION; Heart; endocardium; rheumatic
CHEST; PALPITATION heart
CHEST; PALPITATION heart; lying, while; agg.

Gastrointestinal symptoms

The gastrointestinal tract is also affected in Hirudopatients. It is the part of the body where the greediness of hirudo is expressed mostly. Pains emerge often after eating, esp. overeating. They are not able to give anything, just to take, which might also be expressed by the painful constipation. A lot of cramping and stitching pains in the abdomen, often after eating, are remarkable so as ulcers in the stomach and the abdomen, which might bleed easily.

STOMACH; ULCERS
ABDOMEN; PAIN; cramping, griping
ABDOMEN; PAIN; cramping, griping; morning
ABDOMEN; PAIN; cramping, griping; morning; ten am.
ABDOMEN; ULCERS
ABDOMEN; ULCERS; Duodenum
RECTUM; CONSTIPATION
RECTUM; CONSTIPATION; painful
RECTUM; INFLAMMATION
RECTUM; PAIN; stitching, sharp
RECTUM; PAIN; stitching, sharp; eating; after
RECTUM; PAIN; stitching, sharp; eating; after; one hour after

Symptoms in the female genital tract

In the genital tract cancerous affections of uterus and cervix are remarkable. Once again we see the bleeding tendency in symptoms as leucorrhoea brown, menses too early, menses profuse.

FEMALE; CANCER
FEMALE; CANCER; Uterus
FEMALE; CANCER; Uterus; pre-cancerous
FEMALE; CANCER; Uterus; cervix
FEMALE; CANCER; Uterus; cervix; pre-cancerous
FEMALE; LEUCORRHEA; General
FEMALE; LEUCORRHEA; General; menses; before
FEMALE; LEUCORRHEA; brown
FEMALE; LEUCORRHEA; brown; menses; before

FEMALE; MENOPAUSE
FEMALE; MENSES; General; appear; would appear, as if
FEMALE; MENSES; frequent, too early, too soon
FEMALE; MENSES; late, too
FEMALE; MENSES; painful, dysmenorrhoea
FEMALE; MENSES; profuse
FEMALE; MENSES; scanty

Headaches

The headache is beating and pulsating, which could also be interpreted as a physical expression of the swelling tendency of hirudo.

HEAD; PULSATING, beating, throbbing, forehead

Case boy, 13 years old

General impression of a poor family, not only from the economic side, but also basic concerning a cultural level. The boy seems to be irritated because his parents were talking about him. He did not want to be caressed by his mother. The family tried to do their best but the child did not want it. He suffered from a blood disease, which was very rare. After each accident it could happen that he bleed a lot. Because of nose bleeding he has been already 4 times in hospital. The child wanted to leave the room during the consultation afterwards he got cross. He has a very strong appetite with a big craving for meat. He eats in a strange way. This idea that he must grow is a kind of obsession for him, he is afraid that he could loose energy if he does not get enough, he checks his weight daily. As a younger child he suffered a lot of diarrhoea and there was an allergy against fructose .It was always a problem for him that he could not grow enough. As a young child he grew very quickly, afterwards he stopped growing for years. In the beginning the parents worried about this, afterwards when they stopped worrying the child started worrying about his growth. After the delivery his mother was operated, an extirpation of the uterus, because she had a disease of the placenta. So she was not at home for quite a long time and he was not breastfeed. He did not grow enough; he had an allergy against fructose and a kind of rheumatism after several tonsillitides. Already as a very young child he was fond of meat and his parents were vegetarian. His mother was in the beginning full of resentments towards him because she always wanted to have many children and she considers the child to be in some way responsible for the fact that she has no uterus any more. When the child got ill she was so afraid to loose him. His father said that when the boy arrived their life changed dramatically. The parents described his character as difficult, egoistic, he always thinks of himself. He is so obstinate when he wants something. In school he is always ready to catch something from the others. He has very high expectations towards himself; if he does not succeed he is very cross. He wants to stop studying instead of this he wants to become rich. He is so greedy even at the table. He is never happy and content. Bellyache with cramps is a constant symptom. When the cramps stop he starts eating immediately. He eats much more than he needs. He is fond of meat, butter and spicy food. Everything he drinks must be very cold. His favourite colour is violet; he always wanted to have a violet room. He does not want that somebody looks into his room and he has an aversion against sunlight.

Case, man, 66 years old.

His doctor has sent him, he hates doctors and medicine. It is difficult for him to ask for help, he is a self-made man. He comes from a very poor family. Being well known in the village, he is a kind of gambler, who makes money with it. He appears as a cold, hard person, who has a naughty behaviour, which makes you easily irritated. He is daily at war, like an animal, which lies in wait. He suffers from 2 ulcers on the lower limbs, which started after a motorcycle accident. He had varicosities before. The ulcers were treated in hospital. 2 times he suffered from phlebitis and felt his legs very swollen almost bursting. When he was a child he suffered from a heart disease.

"I do not like doctors and medicine, they just make you loose a lot of money, but probably when medicine costs something I will invest more energy."

The pain in his legs is swelling and bursting, he has the impression as if they would be legs of a hippotamus. He makes the ulcers bleed as most as possible with the idea that then it would be a little less awkward. He feels such a cold inside himself. He has very high blood pressure since years but does not take any medicaments. Years ago he got syphilis "from a bitch". For years he was suffering from ulcera ventriculi et duodeni. He did not realize the pain but started to eat more, the more he was eating the worse it was. He always eats more than he needs he is very greedy.

Having grown up in a very poor family, he always ate more than he needed to have reserves for the next day. One day his stool was black but he did not feel bad at all. He was always drinking very cold water. He suffered from constipation since childhood. A diet did not change anything. He has an aversion against vegetables but just likes to eat meat. What is interesting for him is to feel full. He often had an angina as a child and each time it was related with nose bleeding. He started to work very early because he did not want to go to school any more. He did not play when he was a child but just wanted to play with money. He wanted to grow up as soon as possible to be able to work. He never wanted a companion, he does not trust anybody. He had a wife but they left each other several years ago.

His sleep is quite well but he is tormented by horrible dreams: Once in a dream he had to escape from a truck, which was filled up with some inflammable material. He was in the desert and because of the heat the material could explode every moment. On the other hand he could not escape because there was just desert and he knew the desert would kill him. He is completely photophobic; he loves humid, rainy days.

Common themes of bloodsuckers

- Selfishness
- Taking profit
- Greediness
- Insatisfaction
- Aversion company
- Competition
- Persecution
- Desire for meat
- Chilliness
- Photophobia

Differentialdiagnosis:

Selfishness, taking profit: ***Pediculus***, who has more social contacts than the other bloodsuckers, forces the others to do what he wants by lamenting. Showing the others how needy he is his dictatorial way to make sure that the others stay close to him. **Pulex** takes everything from a person or situation without regard just to taste the experience. Once he has enough he quickly changes," jumps" from one person or situation to the next We also find "jumping personalities" in **Tuberculin** or **Medorrhinum**. In Tuberculinum there is a real desire to exchange experiences with others. Tuberculinum is seeking for contact. Enthusiasm and sympathy, the desire to "get infected with something", qualities which do not appear in pulex, are very important for this remedy. Medorrhinum who also never gets enough wants to be in contact with everybody and wants to experience everything in life." It is a grief that I cannot love all the women in the world". The affection of Medorrhinum is serious. **Hirudo** is more interested in taking profit out of situations, where he sees a possibility for material enrichment. The selfishness in cimex is always related to destructiveness. **Cimex** has awful relationships with other people. To harm somebody else could be a pleasure for him. The loneliness of the bloodsuckers is not perceived as loneliness as e.g. in the drugs. **Drugs** feel all-alone in the universe and they do not have the competitive side of the bloodsuckers. It is much more the selfishness in the bloodsuckers, which causes the fact that they prefer to stay alone.

Insatisfaction: Hirudo has no idea for the right measure; he always takes too much with a strong tendency towards overeating. In pulex there is a constant need for changing situations and partners. Pediculus stays in the same situation but is lamenting .In cimex insatisfaction is expressed by a strong tendency towards destruction and violence.

Competition: Cimex lives his competitive side in a destructive way. "Stealing is my philosophy." Hirudo and pulex are more constructive and have high expectations towards themselves. It is not important to destroy somebody else to be the winner, but if it happens they would do it without regard. In pediculus competition is not so strong than in the other bloodsucker. Competition in the **Labiatae** is completely different. They are much more creative and constructive.

Persecution: Hirudo dreams of having to flee from exploding trucks, from heat, fire and sun. Cimex dreams of having to hide in the toilet with an awful smell. It is also expressed in the delusion that he has to creep into himself he could not sufficiently crouch together. Pediculus has to flee from water.

Swelling attitude, swelling pains: Being insects there is a "swelling" attitude in pulex and cimex but the swelling tendency on a physical level is stronger in pulex. Hirudo fears that he could loose energy so he has to fill himself up with food. It is also expressed by swelling pains, esp. in the lower limbs.

Stitching, burning pains: As stitching and burning pains are typical for insects it is evident that it also comes up in pulex and pediculus.

Itching: Itching is characteristic for pulex, cimex and pediculus reminding us of the animal's bite, which causes intense itching. Itching is not found in hirudo, of which the bite is anaesthetising.

Disgust, offensive secretions: In cimex disgust towards himself and others is more expressed than in the others and it is often combined with violence. But we also find it in pulex and pediculus, whereas in hirudo it is not from importance. The same is valid for offensive secretions.

Bleeding tendency: It is typical for hirudo and not from importance in the other bloodsuckers.

Desire for dark: It is mostly expressed in hirudo, cimex and pediculus.

Chilliness: Considering the chilliness as an expression of emotional coldness it is evident that it is more visible in pulex and hirudo, than in pediculus where emotional contacts are formed easier.

Desire for icy cold water, for wine: The desire for very cold water is typical for pulex, hirudo and pediculus, whereas the desire for wine, which ameliorates symptoms, is seen in cimex and pulex.

Aversion vegetables, fruits: Pediculus and hirudo show the aversion against fruits and vegetables. Hirudo may also have an allergy against fructose.

STIMULANTS

COFFEA CRUDA

Classification

N.O. Rubiacea as Coffea cruda, Coffea tosta, Coffeinum, Ipecacuana, Galium aparine, Mitchella repens, Cahinca, Rubia tinctorum, China officinalis.

Description

Coffea cruda is to be prepared of the seeds of the best Arabian coffee; lesser species were Robusta and Liberia.

It is said that a shepherd, who observed, that animals, that ate some berries, were awake all night long, discovered coffee.

The leaves remain at the tree for three to five years; the blossoms only last for a couple of days. There are berries in different stages of ripping and blossoming at the tree at the same time, all year long.

Traditional use

Early use was to stay awake during night services.

In very early days it was used as a curative in Arabia and the Yemen.

Toxicology/Pharmacy

In Kola, Tea, Guarana and Cacao there is caffeine as well, also in 660 other plants.

Substances in the plant are theophyllin and teein.

Physiologically it is an adenosine antagonist.

Homeopathy

Many symptoms can be found in the rubrics of mind, head (all senses are over-active, very sensitive to impressions and pain, excessive joy can cause all kinds of symptoms) and female (esp. labour pains). There is a strong relationship with toothache, sleep and fever. Out of 1832 symptoms, there are 378 to be found in the mind rubrics, 50 in the rubrics of the teeth, 50 are symptoms of fever and 100 rubrics can be found under female. Remedies like Kava, Kola, Guarana, are stimulants as well. All these remedies have excitement, excessive excitation of the senses and increased activity of the nervous system. Coffea can be differen-tiated in the rubrics sleep, fever and toothache. In pharmacology coffea is used very frequently against headaches – especially migraine

The excitation of all senses cruda is much stronger in Coffea cruda than under Coffea tosta.

Discussion of themes of Coffea

Abuse of, poisoning from
Activity
Anaesthesia/Hyperaesthesia
Ascending agg. (related to mountain sickness of Coca)
Apoplexy, Arteriosclerosis.
As if body would burst.
Bending, turning agg.
Coldness/Congestion-fullness
Convulsions (mostly from emotions, laughing, nervousness, dentition.)
Efficiency increased
Energy, lot of
Exaltation of all powers of the body
Faintness (emotions, laughing... every stimulus is too much or perceived as overwhelming, leading to breakdown)
Food: Wine, coffee and other stimulants
Haemorrhage
Ice, amel. in mouth.
Intoxication, also feeling of intoxication.
Lassitude and inclination to lie down (contrary of exaltation)
Lightness, sensation of

Music agg.

Numbness

Over sensitiveness to allopathic medicine

Pain appearing and disappearing suddenly, like a shock

Pain, torn in pieces, but also many different kinds of pains. Pain is perceived very strongly. All the senses are excited. Pain receptors are sensitive and stimulated by anything - so no evident prevalence of any kind of pain.

Restlessness

Repose amel.

Sensitiveness

Shocks, sensation explosion like flying in pieces

Tobacco, sensitive to

Weakness

OVERSENSITIVITY/OVERREACTION

Coffea perceive and react as if everything around them is too much. In the repertory we see many "ailments from" - similar to what is seen in the rubrics of pain. Every kind of stimulus, also pleasant ones, is perceived as something not able to endure. Even joy is perceived in a distressing way. They cannot withstand any situation that is out of the normal. Objectively the situation is harmless, but they overreact, perceiving this situation as unbearable. To them everything seems to be a shock.

They are very weak persons, have problems with their surroundings, their tolerance level becomes lower and lower. They feel overstressed by the situations they live in; therefore they tend to use all kinds of stimulants, to be able to deal with their daily life. Already without the stimulants they are overexcited.

"I can't live without my morning coffee". By this constant over stimulation they become more and more sensitive und vulnerable. (Drugs don't add new energy to a system, but bring it to a better functioning. Therefore later on they tend to break down, as the system is mentally, emotionally and physically overstressed.

DD Drug-remedies-Stimulants

Drug patients are detached from the world; they try to escape. Coffea uses the stimulants to be able to cope with their situation.

Coffea has many symptoms of anxiety; everything can make him anxious. There are no tears, just anxiety. Coffea cannot bear the idea of suffering, the thought of suffering – he is so oversensitive. Anything that surrounds him is distressing and therefore makes him anxious.

Artificial support

Coffea replaces the support, which is possible to get from other people with a different kind of support, this can be stimulants to help them, or nowadays any medicine. By taking medicines or stimulants Coffea tries to cope with the problem.

To be carried, aversion and desire

Clinging persons or furniture in convulsions

Company, aversion during migraine

Coffea doesn't trust anybody, doesn't believe there can be any help. Mothers for example give painkillers to their children, instead of consoling them. This is a very unemotional help, very typical for today's medicine. There is no difference if they cling to persons or furniture – one as well as the other is only an unemotional object. It is no human or warm relationship – this is similar to the Silica-remedies, they are weak but cannot trust the necessary help and support. Real drug patients withdraw completely, they "fly away", as they don't expect any help anywhere. Coffea seeks for support and help in stimulants. – This is the picture of a lonesome cowboy, far away from home, in the desert, drinking coffee. He is surrounded by dangers, by snakes, native Americans, he cannot ask for help, as there is nobody. He may not sleep, only can stimulate his system to its limits, for to survive in this inhuman surrounding.

On the other side they show up in the practice of the doctor, weeping at every tiny injury. Their emotions are, that this is just the beginning, what terrible experiences will there be in future. Whatever the doctor might say, they can't believe him, as they know that the pain will never stop. Coffea cannot endure the suffering that might come in future. *Ignatia* wants to have attention, and then they feel much better already. This is different with Coffea, Coffea needs medicines, and they cannot trust the human relationship. They feel the best at home with tons of painkillers. Coffea has got a very weak frame; every impression shakes the system and threatens to destroy it. If they can't trust their parents, they can't trust the doctor as well, they only ask for medicines.

<u>Thoughts of death without fear</u>

Like in the **Composite** (as **Arnica, Chamomilla, Millefolium**) there is fear of injuries and in contrast there is the invulnerability of a warrior. **Arnica** sends the doctor home and says he is healthy. As long as Coffea is compensated, they feel omnipotent, when decompensated they are full of anxieties. The delusions of Coffea remind of **Cannabis-indica. Anhalonium** (sees the paradise, is immaterial, of being magnificent, grandeur etc.). Like the true drugs coffea has on one side the feeling of omnipotence and in the contrast the feeling of non-existence. (Feels absolutely alone in the universe, but when able to compensate this, they are the universe. Then it is no longer dangerous to be alone.)

Tries to compensate the feeling of being nothing by an immense productivity, over perfection to feel powerful in some way. If they can compensate perfectly well they get the impression of themselves that they are as good as they would like to be, they feel magnificent, powerful – and this impression of themselves is kind of an exaggeration of their perception. (Nobody can do what I'm doing). Coffea exaggerates the activity until they have a breakdown. The older coffea gets, the more sensitive they become towards the injuries of the world, they loose the power to compensate – and then they get this fear of becoming insane.

Delusion is away from home = wants to be able to close the eyes in a safe surrounding without feeling endangered (the cowboy in the desert, who needs coffee, for not to fall asleep).

Suddenness

Despair with the pains. All the pains appear sudden, like a shock. The suffering is experienced as a sudden invasion. Everything seems to be acute, overwhelming. The despair is huge. Something must happen really fast – they cannot endure it any longer. Menses, dentition can't be stopped; the resentment of what will come drives them crazy. Their own limits must be perceived in these natural processes. Normal physiological processes seem unbearable. They push the system to its limits, to have an apparent safety. Every incidence that might lead them away of their balance is unbearable. They can't trust anybody, can't wait for help of someone. (The strategy of **Silica** is to shrink their environment; I apply only where I'm the best, cut off everything else. Coffea says ok. lets be an over performer, be an omnipotent person, overacting, overdoing. In Silica, the compensation is very different)

144

With the ***drugs*** the problem is a problem of identity, not the problem of being weak and without energy. It is rather the feeling of almost being nothing, probably a kind of depersonalisation. The feeling of isolation is tremendous. In this world no support is possible. They can't trust anybody. Probably there was a kind of environment, where the child was so overprotected by the mother, that it could not develop his own identity, he has only the identity of the mother. So for him the only way to solve this problem is to leave this surroundings and reach another place.

Excitement

In Coffea excitement is not a fundamental but a general theme, a consequence of his state to be. They need to be overexcited to compensate, not to have support. (***Nux vomica*** likes the fight, the argument, wants to show that he is the boss. Like other ***Labiatae*** they have joy in exaltation.)

Fears: Many different fears, as the idea before - every situation can terrify him, everything can be a serious stress. One of the most interesting ones is **fear of killing** and **fear of physician**. The picture of a physician who is taking care of you doesn't exist in Coffea. They can't trust anybody, only in medicine and stimulants. Can't find any support outside of him. **Fear of killing her child** is different to ***Raphanus, Sepia*** and ***Lycopodium*** they are not refusing the child. In Coffea it is more the situation that they want to avoid responsibility.

Coming back to the idea of no support, they had a cold relationship to their parents already. So they can't give on anything different to their child, as they only had experienced this cold relationship. ***Zincum*** is one of many remedies with feeling of weakness, but in Zincum it is an objective lack of power. – Like a car with a lack of gas, that could bring more power, but only has a small amount of gas)

Floating, as if (in different chapters).

Head Pain, from many different stimuli.

Teeth – many problems. Esp. warm things agg.

Sleep – disturbed, by many different things.

Coffea doesn't have a real creativity; it is defence, staying awake, increased efficiency and being on the alert. Studying drug patients, you find many really creative persons, who can't succeed anything. ***Cannabis-indica*** creates wonderful pictures and music. ***China*** only makes many plans, but doesn't realize them.

Nux vomica and *Rhus-tox* are very efficient. *Coca* is used to endure situations with high stress (mountaineering) or to have happy experiences. Coffea is used to stay awake as stimulants, not to be able to work harder or to have supernatural experiences. (*Coca* is one of the most important remedies for cyclothymia)

Coffea - Themes

OVERSENSITIVITY
Artificial support
Suddenness / quickness

Over activity / Restlessness
Over-reacting
Efficiency increased / Alarm (over)

Abuse of drugs/stimulants
Hyperaesthesia
Sleeplessness
Congestion active / apoplexy / fever

Case of Coffea

??- "Before coming to Italy, I have had my thyroid gland checked: I was told, that the left part doesn't work properly and the right part is over functioning. For the last three years I have been taking Iodum."

??-"I have always had problems bottoming my blouse. I had the sensation, that there was something inside, that was blocking, but the first controls did not show anything."

??-"I do not notice any difference ...it hurts a little bit, when I am nervous."

??-"As if it was closed inside."

"My husband says, that I am hysterical, but I call it excitement; I am too excited...."

??-"Whenever there are too many problems, or when the children are sick, or when I have difficulties in getting my work organized...My husband never has such problems, but I do, when I have to organize a day full of obligations. I have always been nervous, when I had to start something new...It may even happen, that I feel blocked on such occasions."

"I happen to wake up without being able to go to sleep again."

??-"I always wake up at three am and at 5 I fall asleep again. Sleep, enough sleep, is essential for my well-being."

??-"I never sleep for 8 hours."

??-"I get aggressive and nervous, because I think that I will not be able to do all I have to do. I try to control myself, but often I just do not have any energy, but with four children this is probably normal. I have had tonsillitis with membranes many times, at least twice a year, I have not had any childhood diseases."

"As a child I have often been afraid not to be able to breathe; I used to call my mother; when I started school I lost this fear. All this stuff doesn't keep me from being a cheerful person. People enjoy my company, because I am entertaining, I am a joker."

??-"I like to eat: fruit, vegetable, fish. Sometimes I really need meat. I have to control my eating otherwise I would be fat. Food is pleasure; I often drink a coffee and I imagine that it helps; I also drink a little cup after dinner, it is my drug.... When drinking tea I cannot sleep."

??-"I remember a frequent dream from my childhood; there was a ball that was growing and growing in size to a point where I was unable to breathe and then I woke up; I was afraid and I did not know where I was. Even now I dream of things that are getting bigger. I cannot explain, why."

??-As a child I often happened to step on people's heels, because I just walked and I did not see people. I was with my thoughts in the sky; I used to be like that as a child, when I was in nursery school; my mother thought it was strange."

??-"It happens to me, when I drive, that I don't pay attention for a minute."

??-"It also happens, that I blush, I hate it ... Also when doing sports my face gets red like a tomato ... I hate people to see it, but there it is, all of a sudden."

??-"My menses are very profuse, frequent and long lasting. Every two weeks and they last for 6 days; I often feel tired; I can have my menses twice a month."

??-"I often suffer from pains in my legs, like stitches...it is as if I was punched and I wake up from the pain...also when I fall asleep sitting on the sofa or while I am cooking... I feel a pain as from a piece of glass."

Therapy: Coffea

Follow-up:

"At first it was horrible, stitches all over my body; it was hard not to drink coffee; only once I had a headache, then nothing, before I used to have them frequently."

??-"Maybe when it is too hot and humid... but after some hours it disappears and it is not so strong as it used to be. I slept better immediately, although I sleep less now. I sleep for 6 hour per day and I am not so tired. I feel fresh and I don´t need coffee any more."

??-" I did not tell you that I have been in hospital to remove a tumour from my right breast; it was three years ago, afterwards I had increasing pains in my nipples.

??-"There, too, I felt stitches coming from outside; it was heavy before menses, but there is nothing now....it is like a miracle; it had started on my left side, then it went to my right side and now it is gone, even when I bump against something....before I was not even able to sleep on my left side..."

??-"I think, it started after iodum. My appetite is normal now, but wine doesn't do me any good...I drink a lot, water or orange juice; I always used to drink a lot, and I love to eat fruit."

??-"I have not been thinking of my blushing... it also appears less (objectively). It is because I am more calm now."

??-"I feel much more quiet and secure about myself... about what I want and what I do not want....it is like that kind of calmness, that I felt on meditating. I feel more secure and decisive."

??-"My menses is normal, much shorter and less profuse...and I don't feel so tired during menses."

??-"In the meantime I have not woken up from the stitches in my legs and even during daytime, I almost don't feel them any more."

Before my mood was very changeable...since my childhood I was always or happy or depressed and now I feel much more balanced. I was very depressed before my menses; I don't have any headaches anymore."

"Anytime I restart my normal life, I feel sad and depressed for some days. then this passes and I try to undertake something; I have to find a rhythm for my everyday life. Also if someone in the family falls ill... I always thought that I was dependant on my thyroid gland."

??-"I don't know where this fear comes from."

??-"I may happen to have some little headaches...for example when the weather is changing...then my head is aching and I get tired. But after one day it is gone."

??-"It starts with my eyes, slowly, slowly, and I have to close my eyes. I must not move... it hurt, when I move my head. But I have had weeks without any headaches."

"The pains in my breasts are completely gone."

??-"Also my weakness is much better.

I feel something in my throat and I don't like to close my blouse. As if something was pushing in the place where I breathe... I have known the feeling since my childhood; I always left my collar open. Whenever I tell fairytales to my children I get the feeling that my voice is failing and it seems weak. As a child I was afraid not to be able to breathe, when going to bed... it was just a sensation, I don't feel this anymore...just in my childhood."

??-"It happens that I eat too much salty stuff ...I know it is not good for my health but I do it many times."

"I have had a strange dream; I remembered that I had it many times when I was a child: I used to dream of a friend, who was dying...I was so sad every time and

I suffered, because I thought it was true; I never knew, whether it was real or imagination."

??-"Now I believe that dreams are another kind of world, but as a child I felt it as an inside world. ..I also dreamed that he was drowning and completely bloated. Once I have seen a drowned person, who also looked very bloated. But this time it did not seem so horrible to me; I simply thought that it was the right moment for my friend to die, who had always wished to dive deep down under the surface of the water...he was a kind of Ikarus of the sea… I was satisfied, because he had decided to let go and I knew it was good for him and for me, too. I knew we would nevertheless always be united, even if he had gone somewhere else now. I felt very touched because it was so beautiful."

PAULLINIA SORBILIS

Synonym: Brazilian Coca, Guarana

Classification

Plantae; Spermatophyta, Angiospermae - Flowering Plants; Dicotyledonae; Rosiflorae / Rosidae; Sapindales; Sapindaceae

Description

Paulinia sorbilis is a climbing shrub It can be found at the Amazonas and took its name from C.F. Paullini, a German medical botanist. The term **Guarana** is derived from the name of a tribe of Indians living between the rivers Parama and Uruguay. Guarana is made from the roasted seeds by powdering them and making a paste with water. The taste is bitter and astringent. In South America it is used very frequently as a stimulant and there are many adressess for it in the internet.

Traditional use

The rainforest tribes have used guarana as a preventative for arteriosclerosis, an effective cardiovascular drug, analgesic, astringent, febrifuge, stimulant and tonic They used to treat diarrhoea, hypertension, migraine, neuralgia, and dysentery. Today the plant is known and used worldwide included as the main ingredient in the "national beverage" of Brazil, "Guarana Soda".

Medicine/Pharmacy/Medicine

Guarana seeds contain caffeine.theophylline and theobromine. It also contains large quantities of tannins, starch, a saponin and resinous substances. The caffeine from Guarana is absorbed in the intestines slowly within 6 hours. In Coffea it is absorbed in the stomach very fast (Guarana contains three times more caffeine than coffee – Coffee stimulates very fast, the Guarana effect stays for over 6 hours, therefore there aren't the sudden Coffea-effects.)
Guarana stops the aggregation of thrombocyts (not the same in Coffea); it is antioxidants, lipolytical and unpoisonous.

Discussion of Paullinia sorbilis themes

Overstimulation/ambition

When Massimo prescribed this remedy he thought of the coffea themes, but the coffea prescription didn't work. Paullinia sorbilis seems to be between Coffea and Coca. Coffea doesn't have very high abilities. Paullinia sorbilis and Coca have the ambition to become better and to reach more; they are very competitive. Coffea tries desperate to reach the normal level.
Desire for abuse of intoxicating substances is much stronger in Paullinia sorbilis. The **artificial support** is more needed to become physically stronger in comparison with Coffea, that needs the stimulation for the mental abilities. It's closer to what we can see in Coca. Paullinia sorbilis seems to be closer to Coca generally. Coffea tries to reach or hold the level others are on. Coca has high demands and strong abilities.
Coca is very egotistical, egocentric. Coffea doesn't trust in anybody, can only trust in pills and stimulants, can't get any energy from friends.

Congestion

In Guarana we see congestions in the chest. It has heart problems and irregular pulse, especially paroxysmal tachycardia; the heart is beating out of control.

They take anabolics to become physically strong. They must become stronger, to be more powerful and competitive, to be able to protect themselves. Paullinia sorbilis is more physically orientated.

Guarana reduces the appetite like amphetamins. They have the feeling of a supernatural energy that allows ignoring all physical needs. Different to Coffea it has problems with constipation, with the urination. All natural and physiological needs can be suppressed.

Feels like a supernatural being, doesn't need to eat, to urinate, to sleep, etc.

DD: *Platina* there is a disgust for all these ordinary human needs – with Paullinia sorbilis there are more these Amphetamin – like sensations)

Other significant characteristics

Feeling of omnipotence, like in all other drug-remedies. Cheerfulness, happiness.

Delusion is about to die (from tuberculosis).

Dreams, women, leprous. Dreams of being a leper.

Excitement, nervous.

Over sensitiveness, in general, like Coffea.

Same excitement like Coffea.

Hilarity, vivacious etc. like Coffea.

Fullness, heaviness and pulsations like in Coffea.

Gen., coffee agg.

Gen., tea agg.

Restlessness.

Sleeplessness

Summary of Paullinia sorbilis themes

Sensitiveness

Over stimulation

Suddenness

Congestions

Ambition

Chest symptoms /tachycardia

KOLA NITIDANS

Plant

Kola is a species of the genus sterculia of the sterculiaceae.
Botanical name: Sterculia acuminata.
It grows in Africa, between Sierra Leone and Congo. It is a small tree, resembling somewhat the chestnut tree, and may attain from ten to twenty feet in height. The fruit of the Kola (the nut) contains from ten to fifteen seeds, chestnut form, and of variable dimensions; these are red or white; the colouring matter is exclusively in the epidermis. The seeds easily separate into two halves, of rosy or white colour. The substance is composed of cells, stuffed with large starch grains, resembling a potato on section. It is in these cells where the caffeine and theobromine are found. The Kola tree bears its nuts when about ten years old. At this epoch a well sized tree may produce eighty or ninety pounds of nuts twice a year.

Traditional use, myths

These are made much use of by the natives, who attribute to them divers medical properties. They are, for instance properly used for their stimulant, sialagogue and stomachic effect. The Africans chew them as much as the Brazilians chews coca, and they ascribe to them quite as marvellous properties. In certain districts of Africa, visited by that daring traveller, Rene Cailie, he found Kola nuts so much prized by the natives as to be used for money. The white Kolas were regarded as valuable presents, e.g. between a host and his guest. To send a person red Kolas, however, was regarded as an insult. Solemn oaths were, in fact, made on the Kola, which was treated as a sort of fetish. Its active principle is caffeine. It also contains Theobromine and Tannin. The powdered nut contains two parts Caffeine.
The Arabs used the nut to reduce thirst and hunger, no caravan left for the desert without Kola nuts.

Proving

By Bernd Schuster that is published as a book.
The following are some of the symptoms of the proving:

Stomach:
'I could just eat and eat.'
'Ravenous hunger, I devour everything without my stomach being full.'
'Enormous appetite, feeling of emptiness in my stomach.'
'After eating I soon feel empty again, and shake'.
'I have to eat something at once'.
'Yesterday I ate lunch twice, then cake and then another hot meal.'
'I feel as if I haven't eaten for weeks.'
'I feel that food is falling into a hole and that my stomach is not being filled at all. I stuff myself with anything I can get hold of. If I do not eat enough I feel nauseous.'
'My blood sugar is low, my whole body starts shaking. Better for eating chocolate.'
'Craving for sweets at 5 pm.'
'I must eat a bar of chocolate to stop the shaking. I think I must get my blood sugar checked.'

Male:
Desire increased
This could also be seen in terms of a sexual appetite (but only in the male provers none of the women had an increased sex drive, though there were three times as many female as male provers). However this male sex drive is more from a feeling of excessive fullness that needs to be discharged than a sense of emptiness that needs to be filled.
'Strong erections in bed without corresponding feelings'
'Insatiable in terms of sex'
'I want to have sex with two women.'
'Intense sexual desire'
'A constant desire for sex'.
'Strong desire for intense sex. I feel I could go on all night.
I still do not feel satisfied after [having sex] twice in succession.
My sex drive is extraordinarily active at the moment.'

'Excessive sexual desire.'

'I think will have to get myself another woman or turn gay, otherwise it till drive me mad.'

'Penis still not flaccid after third orgasm.

'Lecherous thoughts.

Erections with discharge of semen'

'Strong urge to masturbate'

Accompanying symptoms of gonorrhoea:

'A burning on urination, passing thick yellow pus staining the underwear.'

'A constant discharge, unbearable burning when urinating.'

'Squirting off centre flow of urine.

Fullness

is in fact prevalent throughout the whole of the body:

Abdomen:

'My belly is unnaturally swollen and really bloated'.

'Swollen belly after potato soup as if pregnant.'

'Swollen belly which feels like an inflated balloon.'

'Sensation as if I have swallowed a hot ball.'

'I have to undo my trousers because it feels as if the button is pushing into my belly.'

Digestive tract:

'It feels like a balloon was bursting in my abdomen when I pass wind.'

'Severe diarrhoea that comes out in a torrent.'

'I feel as if everything is being emptied out of me. I feel in as if my insides were being turned inside out.'

'Constant urge to defecate but it doesn't provide any relief.'

'Diarrhoea almost spraying out.'

'Strange noise in my abdomen as if a water sluice was being opened. I run to the toilet and it starts shooting out of my anus like a waterfall. I could sit on the toilet the whole time. As soon as I get up I have to go back straight away.'

'Constantly running to the toilet, as soon as I get up from the toilet it starts again'.

Head:

'Feeling as if my skull is too small, as if my brain is expanding.'

'Feeling as if the brain is coming out at the back.'

'Pressure in my head from inside outwards.'

'Ringing headache as if bursting.'

'Feel as if my skull will burst.'

Here we see that because, unlike in the abdomen, there's no outlet in the head, there's a bursting feeling and a sensation of trepanning, of drilling a hole in the head as if to let the pressure out:

'An intense headache as if someone is sticking a needle into my head. The pain feels as if someone is drilling a hole, then poking around with a rod inside my head. Feel as if I can actually take hold of the nail.'

'Feeling as if a nail was being hammered into the middle of the left skullcap.'

Eyes:

'Feeling as if the eyes were under great internal pressure.'

'Feeling of enlargement of the eyes, especially when closing the eyes.'

'Feeling that the intracocular pressure is increased, the eye is getting bigger and is about to burst.'

'Feeling as if the eyeballs have grown.' 'Feels as if my left eye might pop out.'

'Staring, eyes remain fixed on objects. Eyes staring when driving, getting stuck on objects.'

Several provers had sties, and others had eyelids that became oedematous and swollen.

The trepanning sensation is also present here:

'A stabbing pain in the right eye like a red hot needle.'

'There's a violent pain in the right eye as if a blunt object were being pushed from the outside in.'

The only outlet available is lachrymation:

'The pains are > for profuse lachrymation.

Ear

Pressure is also present in the ear symptoms:

'Feeling of pressure in the inner ear, as if the eardrum was bending outwards.'

Feeling of a plug of cotton wool in the ear. (Several provers)

There are lots of whistling noises in the ear. Lots of tinnitus,

'Tinnitus like water rushing in a pipe.'

'Buzzing in the ears like mains electricity or radio.'

'Noises in the ear like the humming of machinery. I've struck my ear several times out of desperation.

Mind

In the Mind section there is a feeling of great potency, ambition and competitiveness like that found in Coca:

I feel full of energy and power. I could carry the whole world on my shoulders. I feel strong and invincible.'

In the evening, strong sexual desire with prolonged erections and a feeling of great potency'

I seem to burn with a big bright flame. A frantic urge to spend in the morning absolutely must have something new. I would really like to buy fantastic things

There is also this same idea of internal pressure:

'Quarrelsome, aggressive, irritable and sensitive.'

'I am very aggressive. At work I behave like a dictator.'

'Sudden weeping.'

'I'm irritated, I feel like a caged tiger.'

'Just a single wrong word makes me explode.'

'I feel like a horse that just neighs, rears up, lashes out. It rolls its eyes and is likely to break loose all of a sudden.'

'I am bursting with energy. I feel hyperactive. Wound up lie a jack in the box. I've got to move, to do something, otherwise I will go crazy.'

'Agitation and tension.'

This pressure finds its outlet in intense activity, particularly work. One prover describes how he was moving house and he picked up all the furniture by himself, running up and down the stairs without getting tired. 'I feel as if I have built up my reserves of energy too much, there's too much energy available.' 'I cannot relax, I work like a mad thing.'

'Strong competitive thoughts. Ambition to be better than others.'

'Able to concentrate well on my work. Worked well, very effectively.'

'Doing twenty things at once, not a moment's rest.'

Violence:

'I'm getting aggressive towards the children who have irritated me in the extreme. I put one out in the cold and rain in his pyjamas. And I nearly crushed the other one's hand, which he threatened me with. During the outburst of feeling I still felt good. I demonstrated my superiority and power. I've never before used physical violence to exert my will.'

'I'm imposing my will on people. I am pushing myself forward. I am better able to assert myself.

Or aggressive sexual behaviour:

'I force my will on a woman and she totally submits. I can do what I want with her.'

'My partner is jealous of a female friend. She annoys me so much with her jealousy that I describe how wildly I had sex with the other woman.'

I mentally undress every woman. I am becoming aware of my charismatic effect on women.

One prover talks about letting off steam:

'I started playing my accordion loudly for 3 hours at home. I always wanted to do it but never did it before. I let off some steam. People did not like it, it was wonderful.'

Another prover says:

'I feel like a pressurized steam sterilizer where the safety valve is blocked. I think I'm going to explode any minute.

Dreams:

In the dreams we see the same themes coming through. There's a theme of very fast motion.

Dreams about sports cars.

Dreams of racing boats.

Dreams of rollerblading

Dreams of cycling.

Strong sexual dreams:

I dreamt of gratifying several women at once.

Dreamt of a group sex scene.

Dreamt I visited a brothel with a friend.

Dreams of a victorious struggle over superior forces: I'm fighting a superior opponent with a sword, in a high-risk building. At the last minute I manage to behead him. Totally exhausted and bleeding, I fall to the floor. My last thought is, I won.

I am fighting a mighty dragon, which as devoured nearly everything that means anything to me. The fight demands everything of me. I smashed the dragon to pieces.

Here we have dream that illustrates the whole theme of a build-up of steam pressure: I woke up because of unusual noises in the cellar. I go to investigate and I find my father, who died nearly ten years ago. He is mentally totally confused, and is dismantling the boiler. As a result, everything heats up. There is too much pressure. There is a risk of explosion. It's like an infernal machine with streaming valves, unfamiliar dials and clocks. In desperation I try to turn down a dial, which is in the danger zone. It's on the red, on the danger level. Danger, everything is blowing up, the ground is shaking, and at the last minute I find the emergency cut-off switch. I wake up agitated.

Another prover had a dream the gas cooker explode in the apartment underneath his own.

In the decompensated state there is the weakness and lethargy typical of all drugs. To be able to understand Kola it is important to compare the group of the drugs to the group of the stimulants. Often we can't make a sharp distinction between both groups. There is a continuum. (***Arum triphyllum*** - Jack in the pulpit - eaten by bears when wake up from their hibernation to shake off lethargy, a mere stimulant).

DD drugs – stimulants:

Themes of the drugs

Isolation / avoidance
Omnipotence / nullipotence
No frame identity
Altered perceptions

Analgesia / Hypersensitive

Space and time
Activity / apathy
Coldness
Music / art / creativity
Transgression (crossing of social borders)

Stimulants are Coffea like remedies. (They react like amphetamines).

Drug like remedies are Cannabis, Laurocerasus, Psilocybe, Coca, Camphora, Penthorum, Nabalus, Agaricus, Opium, Piper methisticum, Bufo, Helleborus, Lithium carbonicum...

Also within the group of the drugs there are big differences, e.g. between Agaricus and Heroin. Drugs were more used to reach spiritual experiences than as a stimulant. We can see that most of the drugs are considered as holy or sacred. Some of these substances are used as drugs as well as stimulants. *Cann-i.* can also be used as a drug to go into a battle, to allow you to feel omnipotent and to kill. But there are some drugs that are much more physically oriented, like *Bufo rana* although it is a hallucinogen (See the fairy-tales connected with toads). With Bufo you don't see the creativity of the drugs, Bufo tries to inflate physically, a common and basic idea of many animals to frighten their enemies when they face a threaten. At the other end *Psylocybe* and *Anhalonium* are real hallucinogenic substances where the attention to the physical world or the own body is not present at all.

A common theme of all the drugs is isolation. They cannot develop an extreme personality, as there is nobody who reflects them. This theme of isolation can be a very useful differentiation between drugs and stimulants, but the differential diagnosis is not always that easy.

Coca has got the typical cyclothymia alteration, being either the prominent winner or the absolute loser. It is difficult to deal with them as a partner, as they always try to prove, that they are the better ones in the relationship. A real contact with other people is hardly possible. The only relationship with people is in their job, like a maniac. An example is one of the best lawyers in a bid Italian city. He is an excessive workaholic and these periods are followed by times of total paralysis. During these episodes of depression he is unable to leave the bed.

Coffea feels isolation as well, but they force their system to have contact with the society. We don´t see the idea of avoidance as in the drug-remedies.

The drugs have actually alternated perception. The surrounding is percept as a delusion. The borders between delusion and reality are vague. Space and time are the base of our limits, if we transgress this frame, we can become insane.

The stimulants hardly ever reach the stages of omnipotence, that we can see with the drugs (hardly ever see themselves as god, devil, Virgin Mary, etc.).

Stimulants are tools to reach the borders within our own limits, not to transgress the human limits and to become superhuman.

There are no strict differentiations between the drugs and the stimulants; Bufo is at the lower end of the drugs and Kola at the upper end of the stimulants. With the drugs we often see analgesia, with the stimulants the opposite, hyperaesthesia. (Morphium is a painkiller and Coffea produces hypersensitivity) Activity and apathy are to be found in both groups, but the drugs show more apathy in the consultation, when compensated, they don't go to the doctor. The stimulants go to the doctor, because they are over excitable and overactive. When treating a drug case, you must be happy if you can help them to compensate, otherwise they might fly away some day, it is not likely that they can be cured. With the stimulants compensation is much more likely.

DD Coca - Kola - Coffea

Kola is on the border between stimulants and drugs. More than Coffea, less than Coca. As Coca belongs to South America, Kola belongs to Africa. Discharging, putting out something is an important idea of Kola. More internal pressure than Coffea, not as sensitive to impressions from outside. More hypertroph, omnipotent, more ambition. Kola feels like a tiger in a cage. They have more feeling of omnipotence or the opposite, the isolation. With Kola there is more the idea of a drug than of a stimulant. It is also harder to differentiate from Coca than from Coffea. Kola is very self-centred; they don't trust the people in their life and show a strong ambition. Kola has got a strong pressure to reach the aim. They are not as phantastic as Coca, aren't so cyclotym, moralistic and single-minded. Kola usually is more successful than Coca. Often they come into the practice, because of a physical symptom. The internal pressure looks for an outlet; on the other side it can destroy them. Kola is dominated by the idea of an energy within themselves, that can tear them apart. Coca has got more the idea of insanity, becoming crazy. Coca is less in contact with reality than Kola. Coffea reacts very strongly to pain, Kola doesn't. Kola seems to be stronger than Coffea. Coffea must stimulate himself, to be able to meet all requirements. Kola is ambitious, has got more feelings of omnipotence.

With the real drugs you hardly ever see some drug abuse. These remedies feel omnipotent out of themselves. They think they don't need any help, neither by anything nor by anyone.

(Omnipotence/isolation). This is mostly seen in Opium, Anhalonium, etc.

EXPLOSION

Kola destroys its company, it doesn't care, what others feel or do, it only needs an outlet for its energy. The physical symptoms show the explosiveness of the remedy (e.g. the diarrhoea). This reminds of **Belladonna** and other Solanaceae. Many symptoms can be seen in both remedies. With chronical Belladonna cases we often get the impression to be dealing with something explosive. This feeling of exploding shows the internal fragmentation, how can one integrate all these pieces to create a whole personality? This feeling that something might explode is very severe, it is a deep problem regarding the own structure. Different pieces are put together in the psyche of a person, to achieve an integer personality. This delusion that one could explode produces enormous fears. (**Baptisia** is already torn apart and tries to put together the components). The drugs don't have an own identity, Kola is afraid to loose the own identity.

Glonoinum, Gunpowder, Aconitum, Ranunculus bulbosus have all this fear of being torn apart. Ranunculus bulbosus is one of the most dependent personalities for M. Mangialavory, you often find drug and alcohol abuse! **Hepar sulfuris** also has got that feeling to explode, to be torn into pieces. The expression of this idea of exploding is always a sign that there is fear one might become scattered in pieces, loose ones own frame. As there are so many symptoms of "exploding" to be found with Kola, this remedy seems to be endangered to loose its identity, its personality.

Like Coffea, Kola tries to stimulate himself, tries to improve his performance.

Dreams of being alone in the world (like the drugs). Sensation of isolation, don't have a real contact with the world. Most likely they did not have a good childhood, no support, the strategy to survive was to show themselves really strong like a macho. Internal emptiness, must therefore constantly overcompensate. Sexuality for example isn't a real contact with a partner, only a kind of masturbation, and a way to get rid of the internal energy; otherwise they become torn in pieces by this energy. Coffea can stimulate himself and then is able to have contact with other people. Kola has to handle energies that actually could destroy him. The disturbance of this system is much deeper.

Falling

Vertigo, same as in Coffea, feeling of being intoxicated. As in many other remedies with the idea of grandiosity the opposite idea of falling is present.

Emptiness / hollowness

Can also be seen with the mushrooms. At the same time there is also the suddenness of the stimulants. Mushrooms grow very fast and collapse fast and easily. **Bovista** is an empty ball that explodes. Here is as well a bad frame of the personality. As with the drugs there were often overwhelming situations in the family. Mushrooms could be regarded as closer to the animals than to the plants. They are like parasites, they transform something.)
Sarsaparilla - Here the emptiness is different. The emptiness is a consequence of a loss, often when they lost someone in the family or a friend. It is as if a part of himself or herself is gone forever with this person).

DD Emptiness in Corallium rubrum:

(*Corallium rubrum* – a sea remedy, needs a very stable environment. Contains a lot of Calcium carbonicum and shows the same weakness. Like Spongia it has got a very simple structure. Is more like Calc-c than like Sil, are very weak personalities that need a lot of support and strong protection. They don't leave the known environment. They cling to one person and don't leave it again – like a coral. The fears of becoming sick are even more prominent than with Calc-c. The example of a child, that grows up with sick grandparents, not with young and vivid parents. They understand very soon that they can die very fast. The child is afraid, the grandparents could die very soon, than it would be alone in the world, without any protection. They don't feel protected enough. They are not actually missing the support; they would need a big rock to feel safe, not only a stone, that won't last forever. They grow up with a big anger. They don't feel enough protected, not valuated; therefore they begin to curse against these imaginary enemies at home. When they had anger at school they come home and swear and curse against the others. This only happens when they are alone. They fight and curse against ghosts; these are the incorporations of those who have hurt him.

A coral for ever stays at the same stone, can't move, has even less movement than an oyster. But it is a bit further in the development than a sponge, as they have got an external skeleton. But they are conscious of the transient protection; the best skeleton doesn't last forever.

Basic personalities hardly differentiated. In psychoanalysis they hardly can reflect about themselves, they can't understand, why something happened.

They have the sensation of a strong internal emptiness (Nicc, Chrom, Pall. They feel hollow, nothing behind the façade).

Black corals aren't corals despite their name. Their skeleton is made out of ceratine. There is a new proving in Italy

PRESSING PAIN

Headaches, many pressing sensations, this is an essential theme with this remedy. With no other compared remedy (neither in Coff. nor in the drug-family), this theme of pressure and the amelioration by discharges (menses, diarrhoea, discharge from the urethra) is as prominent. This is a sign for the danger that the system explodes. They have the sensation that they have to get rid of an internal foreign body. The sensation that they have to stitch a nail through the eye or the head, to relieve the pressure.

Many of somatical symptoms of Cola are connected with the ear, nose, eyes, all possible orifices of the body, as if they could be an opening channel allowing them to discharge something.

Noises in ear

Machinery sounds, echoing, revertebration. These are an expression of a disturbed relationship to oneself. If someone feels like a machine, that is nothing human. With Kola this feeling seems to be very evident. Patients told about this sensation of being a machine, not only that kind of a noise in the ear. Perceive themselves as a machine, like not having a soul, a robot, something not human, just a kind of locomotive.

DD: Collinsonia. - one of the most characteristic symptoms is this feeling that they are a machine.

Discharge

Stomach: Not only ravenous appetite, but a lot of diarrhoea, a lot of discharge. Like an overworking of the digestive tract. That's again the idea of filling themselves with something that can't stay in. Food is felt like an external stuff that has to be discharged as soon as possible, it is not felt as nutrition. Sensation of a ball in the abdomen, they have to get rid of as soon as possible. Only a few symptoms of nausea, but no vomiting, more the direction of diarrhoea. Diarrhoea appears suddenly and disappears suddenly, explosive, gushing, like Coffea. Ravenous appetite - with this input and output.

Bladder: Urging sudden, here again the tendency of getting rid of something.

Sexuality: An apparently more "male" sexuality – "male" is explosive, "female" is implosive. Must get rid of something, not take in something. The expelling in women can be seen in metrorrhagia and leucorrhoea. Metrorrhagia after coition. Orgasm, wanting. (female), doesn't get rid of energy with the intercourse, but takes in some.

Sensation as if about to perspire, but no moisture appears. This is a kind of tenesmus on skin.

So with Kola one can find the themes of Coffea and of the drugs. Very special is this **sensation of an internal pressure, sensation to have to expel something.**

YOHIMBINUM

The themes of Coffea can be used as a working hypothesis for Yohimbinum. Yohimbinum like the other remedies of the Coffea group can be regarded as a stimulant. Coffee usually is used to stay awake; Yohimbinum generally is applied as an aphrodisiac to increase the male potency. With all stimulants the sexual ability is increased, Coffea and related remedies show priapism and sexual overexcite ability, but that is more a side effect of the stimulation of the whole system. The main centre of Yohimbinum seems to be the sexual sphere. The general over stimulation of the whole system as it can be seen in the Coffea related remedies seems to be a side effect in this remedy All stimulants push the system in the direction of omnipotence. This tendency can also be seen in Yohimbinum.

(**DD: Bufo** – we can read in books that they masturbate all day long. But this is only an expression of the general tendency of Bufo, to become swollen, inflated, to be the super macho. There are also women who blow up their appearance, do body building, have their breasts enlarged, etc.)

Many, many symptoms in the rubrics stool, urine and male, also in chest. Flushes of heat (in many organs). Yohimbinum produces burning eruptions and burning pains, reminds of remedies especially like Cantharis, Vespa and other insects. All these remedies also produce congestion in the lower genital region (therefore they also produce inflammation in these regions). These burning sensations and skin irritations cannot be seen in Kola.

Damiana aphrodisiaca. – is very closely related to Yohimbinum. The botanical name is Turnera diffusa. Is also used as an aphrodisiaca, but is not as powerful as Yohimbinum. The symptomatology shows a chronic prostatitis. It does not have as many hallucinogenic symptoms as Yohimbinum, produces more physical problems. Nervous weakness, suppressed and chronic gonorrhoea. Tremendous swelling of the prostate gland and discharges. Injuries of spine.

Over stimulation

Yohimbinum and Guarana were often prescribed when Coffea had not helped. The idea of the over stimulation led to the prescription. Often there were symptoms of Coffea and Cantharis, so the prescription became more difficult. But the **insects** have different central themes than the stimulants. Those patients are more centred on the sexual level. They can have a relationship only by having sex, otherwise they can't feel connected, can't find a protection by the partner. The patients were mainly sent by an andrologist, a friend. Those patients usually have difficulties going to the doctor, as they try to treat themselves with medicine or with mechanical aid, they don't see a psychological background. Coffea as well lives with the perception of its weakness and thinks it only can go into the world if it has taken some medicine that stimulates, psychological help doesn't mean anything for them.

When these Yohimbinum patients had an erection, they were very happy. It was a kind of over stimulation that they tried to reach by injections in the penis or similar remedies. That is a kind of dependence, they enjoy like a junkie. The intercourse itself isn't important, only this artificially produced erection. Yohimbinum has some masturbation as well, but the ejaculation is not important for them, they enjoy seeing their large, erected, strong phallus.

Sleeplessness

In the cases of the four men that were sent by the andrologist sleeplessness started after the beginning of problems with the potency. This began after frustrations at work. They did not feel competent enough in their position as a boss. They had invested all their energy and ambition to reach this position. At the beginning of their career they were highly honoured, powerful men, who did not have any consideration for their private life, to improve their position. They had the choice between their family and their career and decided for the career. As a boss they seemed to be unable to lead a team of colleagues, as they were absolutely self-centred, as they couldn't have a good relationship to their subordinates. Finally they lost their families and failed sexually. The problems with the potency only existed for them in regard of the erection (not ejaculation or orgasm).

Great ambition, but very self centred, not realising that they destroy themselves. It is a very immature, narcistic pleasure. As with the erection they put all their energy in reaching their aim, but cannot keep that what has been reached and perceive that as a total failure. It is this being centred on the idea of the erection, the symbol of a strong man. A failure in this regard is a disaster for their personality. After the prescription the patients often had depressions for months, they were confronted with their shadow.

The patients seemed to be psychologically healthy; they had a perfect façade. It was very difficult to get to know about their problems with other people. They were real workaholics, only interested in their career. (The same with Cantharis – even children are only interested in their career; they want to be the best in class – Verat. as well.).

All the patients had burning sensations or pains, violent diarrhoea, that didn't exhaust them. Whenever they have to do much, they get the diarrhoea.

One of the patients had a strong fear in the youth to be homosexual. He had to prove himself with many women, even horses, that he is heterosexual.

With the Coffea related remedies can be compared: **Damiana. Cacao, Thea sinensis, Chocolade** (seems to resemble Kola in the decompensated level).

They all have problems with children, do not have a deep relationship, and only play a role.

Thea sinensis: The family is a burden. They have problems with emotional matters, can't give them some room. Mostly they are brilliant people, they know what they are doing, and therefore are very successful.

Kola: Is between stimulants and drugs. Very self centred. Have problems to show their insecure side. Like the other members of this group, they do not trust anyone.

Ambition

Very ambitious. On the mental level it is difficult to differentiate it from *Coca*. In Coca the idea of pressure, of pressing pains on the physical level is dominant. Kola does not get lost in delusions as easily as Coca. Typical for Coca is a real cyclothymia; high and low change in short intervals. With Kola these changes are not that prominent, they are more down to earth, more realistic, not so much in their delusion of being omnipotent. So they are more ambitious, more effective than Coca. In Coca there is often an exaggeration of the perception in a positive or negative sense. When Coca does something good, this is fantastic, when it does something wrong, it is terrible. Kola has got more severe depressive periods, is not so biphasic. They work much harder to reach their aims, put much pressure on themselves.

Hypochondria

There is a hypochondriac tendency. The people seem to be strong and fanatic worker (workaholics), are very successful. When they reach their limits, are confronted with health problems, they are shaken. They suddenly cannot rely on their omnipotent system, from now on they decompensate. They become aware of the pressure they are under, and this pressure threatens to destroy them (as if driving a truck with dynamite, that can explode any moment).

Sudden threaten

This idea of a sudden occurrence, a sudden destruction, that extinguishes them forever, can't be seen in Coca. In Coca it is more frequent to the idea of becoming crazy, they become paralysed, cannot move, cannot do anything. They believe so much in their omnipotence, that Thea believe they are immortal. Coca is less related with reality than Kola. If Kola is forced to see a doctor because of a disease, than there are real problems, as they cannot trust any doctor. " Something terrible threatens me, will kill me, and these stupid doctors don't recognize it."

In *Coffea, Guarana* as well as *Kola* there are many symptoms of over excitability. But as Coffea has got strong and exaggerated reactions to all kinds of pain, in Kola one can see more a kind of certainty of a sudden death, that prevents them from reaching their aim. Coffea senses itself weaker than Kola. Kola is much more ambitious. Coffea doesn't want to do too much; they have got enough to do with their momentary duty. They stimulate themselves to hold their achievement, not to reach any aims. They try not to decline in their achievements by taking stimulants. *Coca* is very competitive, as well as Kola and Guarana. *Yohimbinum* is more sexually, male oriented, shows less ambition in regard of reaching a social position.

DD drugs – stimulants:

Usually there is no drug abuse with the drug remedies, in the opposite they are careful about their health and do as much as possible to stay healthy. Because of their feeling of omnipotence they think they don't need anything from outside, they hardly ever take medicine ad only rarely see a doctor. When they allow someone to help them, it is already the beginning of the cure (Opium, Cannabis indica, Psilocybe, etc.). They do a lot to stay healthy, they are almost health fanatics, they don't want to take anything, that might be harmful (drugs, allopathic medicine, etc).

The "amphetamine" remedies are totally different – they have the clear tendency to take too many substances. They seek for a support from the outside. They don't necessarily consume the classical stimulants. Any substance that might support the organism to increase their performance is welcome. A classical example is an American, surfing in the Internet for hours, to find the best "energy-boosting pill", special vitamins, etc.

Coffea tosta

There is an important difference to Coffea cruda; they are seeking for a lot of support. Often first there is a prescription of Pulsatilla, that doesn't work. Shy, timid, almost childish, they need very urgent someone o support them. They are always looking for someone who could take care of them. As Coffea cruda they have got a strong desire for coffee and stimulants, are workaholics, but they want to stay in a safe environment. Very often weak people because of the constant overworking.

Piper metisticum - is much closer to drugs. They have a strong desire to escape from reality. Their situation is not compensated, they can hardly be integrated. Often they are artists or have got an artistic hobby that is very important for them. They need this compensation to endure their normal life. They try in a phosphoric way to live in harmony with others. Often they are ashamed of their artistic abilities. For example the boss of a big company writes poems, fairy tales, etc. It is as if he needs it, to be able to live a "normal" life.

ARGENTUM LIKE REMEDIES

ARGENTUM METALLICUM

Substance

White, soft, shining metal. Argentum is a noble metal, does not react easily with other substances, it is not easily touched by other metals, the less it reacts with others the more it is noble. Aurum is nobler than Argentum, Argentum oxidises, Aurum does not. In capability of conducting electricity and heat silver is better than gold. It is very malleable; in first Rolls Royce argentums was as a transparent film between two glasses, to defrost the glasses. Silver was also used to filter sunlight.

Copper and silver are very often together in nature. It was mixed together first because it makes silver harder and second it doesn't disturb the shining qualities of silver. Sterling silver is a mixture of 92 percent silver and 7.5 percent copper.

Myths/Traditional use

Amalgam is a mixture of silver and mercury.

Used in photography chemistry, because salts of argentum react to light very well.

Argentum is Latin, means shining, reflecting. It reflects over 90 percent of the light, it is useful to filter the water. Holy water also contained silver, and was drunk out of silver cups. Most important enemy of argentum is sulfur, makes it black. The most important enemy of gold is mercury.

Symbolically argentum was related to craziness and to the moon.

Symbolically it is always changing like the moon, shining from the light of somewhere else, strongly related with the night can only shine in the night, also related to the water.

171

In ancient medicine they used water with silver which was exposed to moonlight, amulets with silver, or some other energy which was related to silver to cure mental diseases, which appeared so instable, always changing etc.

There is a strong relation of noble metals to gonads (Platinum, Palladium, Argentum).

Evident connection of the use of these metals and the gonads (in homoeopathy, also in traditional Medicine).

It was used as mirror because it its the most reflecting and shining substance. The moon was related to silver, which is reflecting the sun. Silver is coming from the South American regions, especially Peru. Was related to feminine power and related to the moon. In ancient South American cultures, where they believed in a trinity concept. They considered silver to be negative, gold to be positive and Copper was considered to be neutral, to be a kind of puffer between silver and gold.

In many cultures the moon is related to female, the sun to male, also in alchemy.

If the metals would be parts of a fairy tale Aurum would be the king, Argentum the queen, Platinum the spoiled princess or prince, Cuprum the military part, Sulphur the clerus and Mercury the revolutionary principle.

Sulphur is the greatest danger for the queen (silver which is attacked by sulphur makes it black) and mercury is the greatest danger for the king (mercury is the only substance which is able to destroy gold).

Argentum was used for making money. "Argent" is the French word for money. Only recently we stopped to make coins out of noble metals.

Medicine

Argentum salts are used as disinfectant.

In old surgery it was used as a plating of the tools. They found out if you cut the flesh with a knife plated by silver it is less possible to have infections, because it kills bacteria (they did not know, but the result was much better).

In M. Alzheimer there is a higher concentration of silver in the nerve cells.

What we know about Argentum nitricum homoeopathically belongs much more to the nitricum part than to argentum.

Themes:

There is a strong hypochondriacal tendency especially concerning the mental state and mental diseases. Mental symptoms are over valuated, it is possible that there is a small dullness or dizziness, but it is perceived from this person to be a serious disease. Most of his problems are related to his brain function, to a possible neurological deficit, could be related to delusions of falling out of bed, running against the wall, having an apoplexy etc.

We find an inaccurate judge of distances (running against the wall, delusion floating in the air)

The hypochondriasis is also expressed by rage and fury of having mental diseases and pain. This could finally lead to destruction (suicidal disposition).

A lot of delusions have to do with the ground especially the idea of falling from higher above.

(Del. floating in the air, falling out of bed, mind impulse to jump, vertigo as a fear of falling)

MIND; ANGER, irascibility; tendency; cough; from the

MIND; ANXIETY; fever; during

MIND; ANXIETY; health, about

MIND; ANXIETY; laryngitis, in

MIND; ANXIETY; palpitation; with

MIND; ANXIETY; stomach; in

MIND; CARES, worries; full of; laryngitis, in

MIND; DELUSIONS, imaginations; apoplexy, he has

MIND; DELUSIONS, imaginations; runs; against something

MIND; EXCITEMENT, excitable; tendency; pain, during

MIND; FEAR; apoplexy, of

MIND; FEAR; concussion, of, as if he might run against something

MIND; FEAR; insanity, of losing his reason

MIND; HYPOCHONDRIASIS

MIND; IDEAS; deficiency of

MIND; RAGE, fury; convulsions, fits; after

MIND; RAGE, fury; convulsions, fits; after; epileptic

MIND; RAGE, fury; pain, from

If we combine the idea of loosing the mental ability and the idea of falling from higher above we find one of the main themes of argentum:

Fear of loosing self-control, mental ability, what also mean loosing a powerful position, expressed by the idea of falling. Symbolically talking it could mean to loose the power as a queen (if we consider Aurum being the king and Argentum the queen, as argentum is related to the feminine aspects of life, to the moon, the water)

We have to do with a very clever person, who has this fear of loosing his mental power. Very often there is a great difference between the objective grade of mental deficiency and their subjective impression, they over evaluate their mental deficiency, it is much more the fear that it could be a deficiency. There is a great fear of loosing self-control, of becoming mad, as if there was a severe split in the personality. Often decompensate in menopause or andropause *(ailments from climacteric period)*. Loosing his power, decompensating is very threatening for these persons. It is often mentioned in materia medica for old people but it could also be used for young people, but it is more common to feel that you are loosing your power when you become old.

MIND; SELF-CONTROL

MIND; SELF-CONTROL; loss of

MIND; SELF-CONTROL; wants to control himself

MIND; HANDLE things anymore, cannot, overwhelmed by stress

MIND; HANDLE things anymore, cannot, overwhelmed by stress; fast, when happening fast

MIND; SENSES; control imperfect

Fear of loosing position may also be expressed by

Vertigo

Fear of high places,

Fear of mountains,

Fear of places. (Anxiety walking in open air, could possibly mean the projection of emptiness he fears in himself, or the place where he has to show his self-control to the others)

Fear of buildings (Palladium in architecture, open structure empty inside, very high)

Patients often dream of walking inside of these buildings there is nothing inside, but air (*anxiety in open air agg*) show a beautiful palace but the fear that there is nothing inside.

GENERALITIES; ROOM; agg.
GENERALITIES; ROOM; agg. People, full of

Often in noble metals, somatically talking it is seen as vertigo, fear of falling, mentally talking fear of loosing the powerful position, fear of mountains: They could go in their active life to the mountains, just to prove themselves that they are able to do this.

Idea of *fear of open space* is a common matter for all noble metals, (Arg. Aur, Cupr, Plat) for them open space is a clear representation of something which is bigger than themselves.

A mountaineer who reaches the top, and he is still with the same problems.

"My goal is done, but I have the feeling that it is not reached, but there is nothing left to do, the only possibility left is to jump down ("mind impulse to jump") which could express the suicidal tendency which is also seen in Argentum. (not in the repertory, just argent nitr)

MIND; ANGUISH; clothing too tight when walking in open air, as if
MIND; ANGUISH; walking; air, in open
MIND; ANXIETY; air; open, in; agg.
MIND; ANXIETY; walking; while; air; open, in; agg.
HEAD; EMPTY, hollow sensation
HEAD PAIN; GENERAL; air; open; agg.
MIND Fear of high places (phenix)
GENERALITIES; EMPTINESS, hollow sensation
Vertigo symptoms

Overrepresentation of superego, high expectations towards themselves
There is a very high superego, it could be a child for example playing football, who has to be the captain, if he feels he did not do it well enough it is a disaster for him.

"I had a job to do and I failed." It is a big problem for them; they get easily depressed.

Argentum and also the other noble metals feel a kind of commitment in them, they have to fulfil. If they fail and do not reach their goal it is like loosing the reason of their existence on this planet, which could end in a big depression with a strong suicidal tendency.

The judgement if they were good enough always comes from their own super-ego; it is not so much important how other people think about that.

In **Platin, Palladium and Cuprum** the appreciation has to come more from outside (*desire to be flattered*). If Argentum or Aurum feels that they are flattered not for the right reason they are rather irritated. When they think that they do not deserve the estimation in their opinion they cannot accept it. Often they express the feeling that they are not enough appreciated. It is important which part of the person is not enough appreciated. Aurum, Cuprum, Calcium sulph want to be appreciated in a very different way. For instance **Platinum** believes he deserves appreciation because this is his birthright and is very irritated if he does not get this appreciation. Because I am the son or daughter of the king I have to be estimated. It is my blood; I don't have to do anything for this.

Aurum, **Argentum** think that they have to deserve their appreciation, don't wait to be honoured, but have to do something to deserve it. Then they like and need appreciation of their surrounding. Always put their goal very high. If they really reach the top of the mountain and they cannot get higher they often get their crisis.

They always have a kind of commitment; have to take responsibility for others (like kings and queens are supposed to do).

DD: **Cuprum** wants to be a well-known soldier, would not like to be the king, they compete on a physical level. Argentum competes on an intellectual level and is very affected if he does not reach his own high expectations.

Argentum how it could be seen in children:

Often they belong to demanding families, or more often to families where there was a derangement, for instance. An important family member was a star and fell down; the child has to take care of this to be able to raise the family to the same level as before. We see a strong sense of responsibility, not revolutionary as Mercury.

Need of one good companion on their side

Argentum has to have a strong companion, not somebody, but a powerful person, a need to exchange, not like **Calcium** who needs somebody. Really trust in other people, not so dictatorial as Aurum could be. Faithful persons.

MIND, TALK, talking, talks; desires to, to some one

MIND; TALK, talking, talks; indisposed to, desire to be silent, taciturn

MIND; TALK, talking, talks; indisposed to, desire to be silent, taciturn; company, in

DD: *Arg. nitricum* needs much more somebody very strong who is supporting him.

Aurum needs to be in the centre, must be the chief, has a court around him, has to be sure that he can trust in them. Must be sure that he is adored, well considered, needs more than one person, needs to have friends who are honest, who don't flatter them. In Aurum there is the belief that "I am always alone in my decision, I have the last word alone"

Platinum always has somebody beside him who is very intelligent, a star, whom he cannot reach, but has to jump over him, I cannot reach your point I'm not so intelligent, famous as you but I will show that you are really nothing". Often they use a dominant destroying sexuality for their means. Platinum's kind of competition is to crush the other person down. A spoiled princess/prince. Often they are just interested in sex because it is their way to dominate the other person. When they think they succeeded there is no sexual interest left. More often we find frigidity in platinum then real increased sexual desire.

Sensation of enlargement and constriction

A common theme of the noble metals is an enlarged feeling, which has not only to do with physical symptoms, but with the mental state of being enlarged. The feeling of being the king or the queen, of being a great person, of having a certain social responsibility, of having a commitment in this world. This sensation of being enlarged is related to constriction in Argentum. If something is enlarged it gets easily too tight. *(Del. clothing is too tight)*. Constriction is also very important on a symbolical level.

In Argentum there is the same kind of commitment as in Aurum but unfortunately I am a female, the queen. I have to use a different kind of energy to reach my goal. In history ancient queens were really warriors (aurum quality). Argentum cannot use the somatic attitude to reach the goal but only the intellectual attitude. "I know I have to do something very important I have the same commitment as Aurum but by nature I have not the same tool. So I have to rely completely on my intellect, and the main problem is that I am seriously in trouble to loose my intellect because this is my only tool."

Aurum can trust more in his tools he has more of them. Argentum is insecure about the success of his doing. Nevertheless they have the same kind of commitment.

MIND; ANXIETY; clothing; tight, as if too, walking out doors
MIND; DELUSIONS, imaginations; clothing, clothes; tight, too
MIND; DELUSIONS, imaginations; floating in air
HEAD; CONSTRICTION
HEAD; CONSTRICTION; band or hoop
HEAD PAIN; GENERAL; hat, from pressure
FACE; LARGE, sensation of being
GENERALITIES; CONSTRICTION; internal, sensation of
GENERALITIES; CONSTRICTION; internal, sensation of
GENERALITIES; PRESSURE; agg.
GENERALITIES; PRESSURE; agg.; hat, of
GENERALITIES; PRESSURE; amel.
GENERALITIES; CLOTHING; tight, as if too
FEMALE; ENLARGED; Ovaries
FEMALE; ENLARGED; Ovaries; sensation
FEMALE; ENLARGED; Ovaries; sensation; left
FEMALE; ENLARGED; Uterus

Hurriedness

Argentum must do the things as quickly as possible, because of this growing fear that the brain pathology could make the person unable to work, is not restless but rather quick, must arrive in time (not so restless as in *Zincum* or spiders) this is not seen in Aurum. Aurum has not the fear of becoming crazy.
The fear of anticipation in Argentum is not so strong as in Argentum nitricum.

MIND; HURRY, haste; tendency
MIND; TALK, talking, talks; hasty
MIND; TIME; passes too slowly, appears longer
MIND; RESTLESSNESS, nervousness; tendency
MIND; RESTLESSNESS, nervousness; tendency; night
MIND; RESTLESSNESS, nervousness; tendency; bed; driving out of

Changeable alternating states, esp. on the mental level.
Relation to water, water agg.

As Argentum in many cultures is related to the moon which is always changing and was used in traditional medicine to treat madness which also meant constantly changing states Argentum has also changing states esp. mental states as a remedy.

Possibly these changing moods and states are experienced to be threatening to the mental integrity of the person. If you are not sure about the constancy of your mental ability you will always fear that the alternation, the change could come immediately, makes you mad, stupid, dizzy etc.

The rubrics *"eye looking moving things flowing water agg"*;*"vertigo looking at running water"* could also express the fear of changing states as water is always changing.

MIND; LOQUACITY; alternating with; sadness
MIND; LOQUACITY; changing quickly from one subject to another
MIND; MANIA, madness; alternating with; sadness
MIND; MOOD; alternating
MIND; MOOD; changeable, variable
MIND; WEEPING, tearful mood; tendency; alternating with; cheerfulness
MIND; WEEPING, tearful mood; tendency; alternating with; irritability
EYE; LOOKING; moving things, flowing water, at; agg.
VERTIGO; LOOKING; water, at running
GENERALITIES; WATER; running water agg, seeing or hearing

Loss of brain functions
Often the loss of brain function is perceived more subjectively than objectively, it could be difficult concentration, confusion, dementia, insanity, and mania. Possibly the rubrics *"makes gestures grasping or reaching at something or one spot"* are an expression of a mental disease too.

MIND; CONCENTRATION; difficult
MIND; CONCENTRATION; difficult; afternoon
MIND; CONFUSION of mind
MIND; CONFUSION of mind; intoxicated, as if
MIND; CONFUSION of mind; old people, in
MIND; DEMENTIA
MIND; DEMENTIA; old people, in
MIND; DULLNESS, sluggishness, difficulty of thinking and comprehending

MIND; DULLNESS, sluggishness, difficulty of thinking and comprehending; alcohol, from

MIND; GESTURES, makes; grasping or reaching at something

MIND; GESTURES, makes; grasping or reaching at something; picks at; nose and lips or one spot

MIND; GESTURES, makes; grasping or reaching at something; picks at; nose and lips or one spot; bleed, until they

MIND; IMBECILITY

MIND; INSANITY, madness

MIND; MANIA, madness

MIND; MANIA, madness; alternating with; sadness

MIND; MANIA, madness; rage, with

MIND; MEMORY; weakness, loss of

MIND; MEMORY; weakness, loss of; said, for what has

MIND; MEMORY; weakness, loss of; say, for what he is about to

MIND; MENTAL exertion; agg.

MIND; PROSTRATION of mind, mental exhaustion, brain fag

MIND; PROSTRATION of mind, mental exhaustion, brain fag; morning

MIND; SENSES; control imperfect

MIND; SENSES; control imperfect; sitting or reflecting, also when

MIND; STUPEFACTION,

MIND; STUPEFACTION, as if intoxicated; vertigo; during

Destructiveness, suicidal disposition

If they do not reach their goal in the sense they had expected it or if a mental disease, a pain

Comes up Argentum can be destructive like Aurum. This could even lead to a suicidal tendency. It is not so well expressed for Argentum in the repertory (just Aurum and Arg nitr.)

It could also be expressed physically by destruction of bones, cartilages, cancer, and ulcers.

MIND; RAGE, fury; convulsions, fits; after

MIND; RAGE, fury; convulsions, fits; after; epileptic

MIND; RAGE, fury; pain, from

GENERALITIES; CANCEROUS affections; scirrhus

DD pain in comparison with *Calcium carbonicum*

The pain in Calcium is related to something unknown, threatening because it is so unknown, lives in his shell. Could be any pain, everything is painful and threatening in the same way, childish remedy, has to be protected, supported. In Calc. every pain could be threatening for life itself.

The pain of metals is related with loosing the position, power. Not at all in Calc. Calc is seeking for a parent, a strong personality. Aurum and Argentum are seeking for the few friends they could trust, somebody who could continue the kingdom, don't need a stronger person need equal persons in whom they can trust, who could understand them. It is not any pain like in Calcium; it is more the mental diseases. Destruction and suicide is not at all found in Calcium.

Strong sense of responsibility

Comparable with Aurum, but it is not represented in the repertory.

Fear of snakes

VISION; SNAKE before the vision

Physical symptoms

Vertigo

Vertigo is related to the fear of falling to the fear of loosing position to the fear of failure.

Other symptoms are combined with vertigo for instance headache, loss of vision.

VERTIGO; HEADACHE; during
VERTIGO; HEAT; during
VERTIGO; LOOKING; water, at running
VERTIGO; NAUSEA; with
VERTIGO; SITTING, while; agg.
VERTIGO; SLEEPINESS; with
VERTIGO; TURNING; on; agg.
VERTIGO; VISION, with obscurity of
EYE; CLOSE; involuntary; vertigo, during

Head pain

A lot of pressing pains, which express on a physical level the enlargement and constriction. Head pain with hollow sensation reminds of the fear of buildings with nothing inside. Aggravation in open air as on the mental level.

A violent pain, as an expression of hypochondriasis, is complaining a lot about pains.

HEAD; CONSTRICTION
HEAD; CONSTRICTION; band or
HEAD; EMPTY, hollow sensation
HEAD PAIN; GENERAL; air; open; agg.
HEAD PAIN; GENERAL; binding; head; amel
HEAD PAIN; GENERAL; hat, from pressure of
HEAD PAIN; CRUSHED, as if shattered, beaten to pieces
HEAD PAIN; SQUEEZED or jammed, as if compression in
HEAD PAIN; SQUEEZED or jammed, as if compression in; Temples

Eyes
Very often represented in the repertory is putrid eye inflammation, also in infants.
Further paralysis of optic nerve, concerning once again a loss of brain function, of self-control. Also represented in many blindness symptoms, loss of vision.
Symptoms combined with vertigo. Fear of snakes expressed as "snakes before vision".

EYE; CLOSE; involuntary; vertigo, during
EYE; DISCHARGES of mucus or pus
EYE; DISCHARGES of mucus or pus; purulent
EYE; DISCOLORATION; redness
EYE; DISCOLORATION; redness; headache; during
EYE; DISCOLORATION; redness; lids
EYE; INFLAMMATION; children, infants, in
EYE; LOOKING; moving things, flowing water, at; agg.
EYE; OPEN lids; unable to
EYE; PARALYSIS of; optic nerve, amaurosis
EYE; CLOSE; involuntary; vertigo, during
EYE; DISCHARGES of mucus or pus
EYE; DISCHARGES of mucus or pus; purulent
EYE; DISCOLORATION; redness
EYE; DISCOLORATION; redness; headache; during
EYE; DISCOLORATION; redness; lids

EYE; INFLAMMATION; children, infants, in
EYE; LOOKING; moving things, flowing water, at; agg.
EYE; OPEN lids; unable to
EYE; PARALYSIS of; optic nerve, amaurosis
VISION; DIM; vertigo; during
VISION; LOSS of vision, blindness
VISION; LOSS of vision, blindness; transient
VISION; LOSS of vision, blindness; vanishing of sight
VISION; SNAKE before the vision

Ear

A lot of itching, tinnitus combined with vertigo, many different ear pains.
EAR; ITCHING in
EAR; ITCHING in
EAR; NOISES in

Abdomen

Many different pain symptoms (over 60 in the repertory) expression of hypochondriasis rectum, diarrhoea from excitement as in Arg. nitricum.

Male genitals

One of the main body regions which are affected in Argentum (in other noble
metals as well) are the gonads. Their Argentum shows its destructive side expressed by cancer, tumours, ulceration of mainly gonads, but penis, uterus as
well.

MALE; CANCER
MALE; CANCER; Testes
MALE; INDURATION; Testes
MALE; INDURATION; Testes; right
MALE; TUMOR; Testes
MALE; ULCERS
MALE; ULCERS; Penis
MALE; ULCERS; Penis; prepuce

As in most of the other body regions we find many pain symptoms, violent
pains

And also the symptoms "pain testes, pressure of clothing agg" which expresses the sensation of enlargement and constriction in the gonades, one of the most affected body region.

Inflammation of testes.

Sexual desire seems to be diminished, tendency to impotency. (Argentum cannot really rely on his physical tools)

MALE; PAIN; General; spermatic cords
MALE; PAIN; General; testes; pressure of clothing agg.
MALE; PAIN; General; testes; walking, while
MALE; PAIN; crushed; testes; right, while walking
MALE; ERECTIONS, troublesome; wanting, impotency
MALE; INFLAMMATION
MALE; INFLAMMATION; Testes, orchitis
MALE; SEXUAL; desire; increased; erections; without
MALE; SEXUAL; desire; wanting

Female genitals

As in male gonads strong tendency to cancer, tumours, ulcers and inflammation of gonads but also other genital parts. Enlarged sensation in ovaries and uterus. Many pain symptoms.

Leucorrhoea once again mostly thick, profuse, yellow.

Sexual desire diminished

FEMALE; CANCER
FEMALE; CANCER; Uterus
FEMALE; ENLARGED; Ovaries
FEMALE; ENLARGED; Ovaries; sensation
FEMALE; ENLARGED; Uterus
FEMALE; HARDNESS; Ovaries
FEMALE; INDURATION; Ovaries
FEMALE; INDURATION; Uterus
FEMALE; INFLAMMATION; Ovaries
FEMALE; INFLAMMATION; Ovaries; tubes, fallopian, salpingitis
FEMALE; INFLAMMATION; Vagina; bartholins gland
FEMALE; LEUCORRHEA; profuse
FEMALE; LEUCORRHEA; yellow

FEMALE; TUMORS; Ovaries
FEMALE; ULCERS; Uterus and region of
FEMALE; ULCERS; Uterus and region of; cervix

Larynx and voice

This body region is also strongly affected by Argentum; we find more than 70 symptoms in the repertory.

Once again general features of Argentum are expressed in this body part, as constriction, a lot of pains, destruction (necrosis of the cartilage of larynx).

Inflammation, hoarseness, loss of voice, in singers, overuse of voice, talking agg. On the mental level there could be a connection to symptoms as "desire to be silent in company" perhaps associated to feelings as fear of failure, fear of loosing control, or position.

As an expression of the tendency to neurological disease there is the symptom of "larynx paralysis of"

MIND; TALK, talking, talks; indisposed to, desire to be silent, taciturn; company, in

MIND; FEAR; speak; to
LARYNX & TRACHEA; CONSTRICTION
LARYNX & TRACHEA; FOREIGN substance, sensation;
LARYNX & TRACHEA; INFLAMMATION; Larynx
LARYNX & TRACHEA; INFLAMMATION; Larynx; singers, in
LARYNX & TRACHEA; PARALYSIS
LARYNX & TRACHEA; ROUGHNESS; Larynx; talking, after
LARYNX & TRACHEA; TUBERCULOSIS; Larynx; singers and public speakers
LARYNX & TRACHEA; ULCERATION
LARYNX & TRACHEA; ULCERATION; Larynx
SPEECH & VOICE; VOICE; changeable
SPEECH & VOICE; VOICE; hoarseness; overuse of the voice
SPEECH & VOICE; VOICE; hoarseness; singing, from; agg.
SPEECH & VOICE; VOICE; lost; overuse of

Bones, cartilage

Very strong relation to destruction of cartilages and bones, deforming processes, cancerous processes, chronic inflammation.

Rubrics:
BACK; CARIES, necrosis of; spine
BACK; CARIES, necrosis of; spine
GENERALITIES; BONES, complaints of; syphilitic
GENERALITIES; BONES, complaints of; condyles
GENERALITIES; CARIES, necrosis of; bone
GENERALITIES; CARIES, necrosis of; joints
GENERALITIES; CARTILAGES, complaints of
GENERALITIES; CARTILAGES, complaints of; lesions, syphilitic
GENERALITIES; INDURATIONS; Cartilages
GENERALITIES; INFLAMMATION; bones, osteitis
GENERALITIES; INFLAMMATION; bones, osteitis; osteomyelitis
GENERALITIES; INFLAMMATION; cartilages, chondritis, perichondritis
GENERALITIES; NECROSIS; bones
GENERALITIES; NECROSIS; cartilages

Suddenness

Pains or other symptoms generally appear suddenly or increase gradually and disappear suddenly.

HEAD PAIN; GENERAL; increasing gradually; ceasing suddenly, but
HEAD PAIN; GENERAL; sudden pains
HEAD PAIN; GENERAL; sudden pains; go suddenly, and
HEAD PAIN; DRAWING; Sides; increases gradually and ceases suddenly, feeling as if a nerve had been torn
FACE; PAIN; General, aching, prosopalgia; increasing; gradually and decreasing; suddenly
FACE; PAIN; tearing; increases gradually and ceases suddenly
STOMACH; PAIN; General; appears gradually and disappears; suddenly
CHEST; PAIN; cutting, sudden sharp pain
CHEST; PAIN; cutting, sudden sharp pain; bending forward; agg.
CHEST; PAIN; cutting, sudden sharp pain; respiration, during
CHEST; PAIN; cutting, sudden sharp pain; costal cartilages of short ribs
CHEST; PAIN; cutting, sudden sharp pain; sides
CHEST; PAIN; cutting, sudden sharp pain; sides; left
GENERALITIES; PAIN; General; appear suddenly

GENERALITIES; WEAKNESS, enervation, exhaustion, prostration, infirmity; sudden

One spot
Symptoms or sensations occur in spots.

MIND; GESTURES, makes; grasping or reaching at something; picks at; nose and lips or one spot
THROAT; PAIN; General; spot, in a
LARYNX & TRACHEA; COLDNESS; sensation of, Larynx; spot
CHILL; ICY coldness; spots, in single
SKIN; COLDNESS; icy; spots, in
SKIN; COLDNESS; spots
GENERALITIES; PAIN; General; spots, in small
GENERALITIES; SPOTS, symptoms or sensations occur in

Sensation of foreign body
In several body parts we find sensation as if from a foreign body. (Larynx, head, mouth) Perhaps this sensation is related to the fear of loosing control. If there is something inside a person that doesn't belong to her it makes the person insecure concerning the control about herself.

HEAD PAIN; FOREIGN BODY, as if
HEAD PAIN; FOREIGN BODY, as if; Occiput
MOUTH; FOREIGN body on, as if; Palate
LARYNX & TRACHEA; FOREIGN substance, sensation; Larynx
COUGH; FOREIGN body, as of; larynx, in

Summary:

The most important features of Argentum metallicum are:

Mental level:

Fear of loosing self-control, of loosing mental abilities.
Also real loss of mental abilities as confusion, dullness, madness etc. that is usually much more perceived subjectively than objectively.
Fear of loosing a powerful position, fear of high places.
Hypochondriasis in general but esp. concerning mental abilities.

Overrepresentation of superego, high expectation towards themselves.

Feeling of having a kind of commitment, strong social responsibility.

Need of a good companion on his side.

Hurries have to do their work quickly because there could not be so much time left because of the impending mental disease.

Changing, alternating states esp. on the mental level.

Relation to water, moving objects, which agg.

Sensation of enlargement and constriction.

Destructive tendency seen as severe depression and suicidal tendency when they could not reach their goal, their own expectations. Destructive tendency also on the physical level as cancer of gonads, caries, destruction of bones and cartilages.

Physical level:

Physical parts that are mostly concerned are:

Vertigo: physical expression of fear of loosing powerful position, of falling down.

Head pains: mostly pressing, hollow sensation.

Bones, cartilages: strong tendency to destruction of bones and cartilages. (Cancer, chronic inflammation).

Gonads: cancer, chronic inflammation.

Eyes: putrid inflammation of eyes, blindness.

Larynx, voice: inflammation, hoarseness, destruction of cartilage, and loss of voice.

Chest, abdomen: many pain symptoms, as expression of hypochondria tendency.

Suddenness of symptoms, sudden pains, violent pains, sensitive to pain.

CITRUS VULGARIS

Family

Rutaceae

In the family of Rutaceae 900 species in 150 genera are found in tropical and temperate regions especially in southern Africa and Australia.
This family is the source of some phototoxic chemical compounds.

Citrus

12 species are native to southern China, Southeast Asia and Indo-Malaysia.
Citrus vulgaris synonymes : Citrus Bigaradia. Citrus aurantium amara. Bigaradier. Bigarade Orange. Bitter Orange. Seville Orange. (Sweet) Portugal Orange. China Orange. Citrus dulcis
Flowers large, pure white, strongly scented, bisexual; stamens 15 to 30. Fruit globose, often depressed 6 to 10 cm.
In homeopathy the used part is the fresh fruit peel (with oil glands which are present below the epidermis).
Both common and official names are derived from the Sanskrit nagaranga through the Arabic naranj.
The first mention of oranges appears in the writings of Arabs, the time and manner of their first cultivation in Europe being uncertain.
The small, immature fruits are sometimes used under the name of Orange berries for flavouring Curacao. They are the size of a cherry and dark greyish-brown in colour. Formerly an essence was extracted from them.
The peel is used both fresh and dried. Much is imported from Malta, cut more thinly than that prepared in England.
Orange pickers suffer pricks and scratches from the thorns of the plant and secondary infection. In growing oranges, dermatitis and paronychia due to citrus oils and juices occurs.

Cheilitis and stomatitis were reported from eating oranges. Persons who suck citrus fruits can develop circumoral dermatitis and hyper pigmentation. Cheilitis was attributed to the volatile oil of oranges. Many authors reported dermatitis of the hands from oranges

Anaphylactic reaction from ingestion of orange was reported.

There was found an interrelation between Balsam of Peru and orange peel.

Medicinal action and uses

The oil is used chiefly as a flavouring agent, but may be used in the same way as oil of turpentine in chronic bronchitis. It is non-irritant to the kidneys and pleasant to take.

On the Continent an infusion of dried flowers is used as a mild nervous stimulant.

The powdered Bitter Orange peel should be dried over freshly burnt lime

In Germany the name Zitronenholz has been much more widely applied. It seems to have referred mainly to satinwoods with a lemon scent that were probably responsible for most if not all the reported cases of Zitronenholz dermatitis.

Case of Citrus vulgaris

At the time of the consultation Oreste was a 40-year-old man. Showing at my studio with his wife, he appeared quite anxious. Despite their house was very close, they reached my studio 30 minutes before the fixed time. The patient spoke in tones of emotion, often looking at his wife as if he were asking confirmation of his words. As soon as he sat down, he literally unloaded a thick lot of laboratory exams and medical reports. It was as if he were very concerned with my attention to his case. The reason of his visit was a Paget disease, which had been diagnosed 5 years before, after a long period during which the patient had been showing upper limbs and rachitic pains. In absence of pains at inferior limbs, the raise of alkaline phosphatasis and hydrossiprolinuria were the main pieces of information allowing the possible diagnosis.

Radiography showed that the dorsal and cervical rachitic as well as both the humeri were interested by the disease. At that time a specialised medical centre was following Oreste's case where he used to go at least three times a year.

According to my colleagues' reports, the pathology had become stable: at the time of our interview the patient was not showing pain in his rhachis anymore, and he had been treated with C-vitamin. Anyway humoral exams were still altered. The patient and his wife were running quite a big drugstore. I got informed about the first steps of his disease:

"First Paget symptoms showed with cramps in my arms and in particular in my wrists and further with a backache (dorsal and cervical rhachis)"

I asked whether he could report more precisely:

"I would feel better if I changed my posture and spent my time making outdoor activities. I needed staying in the open air. You know, I am that sort of person who needs keeping in movement ... but, as you know, this disease is not curable"

My main problem, apart from Paget disease, is diarrhoea. Since I was a child I had problems with my intestine and I have diarrhoea quite often, when I get nervous most frequently. I realised I had this terrible disease by chance and I am quite worried for my future and for my old age: I am quite worried on the fact that I might get seriously sick and of not being self-sufficient anymore".

I noticed Oreste was very agitated while he was speaking, as if he were anxious of telling me many things without having the actual time to inform me of everything. He spoke very quickly and after a short time he asked me if he could go to the lavatory.

When he came back he apologised and said: "I am a slave of diarrhoea. I cannot reach a place if I am not absolutely sure there is a toilet available. Also when I enter a tearoom I must be sure there is a free lavatory and that I do not have to wait to enter"

I asked for further information:

"I am always in a terrible hurry, I can't even stand to have to wait for my further breath ...I cannot manage to do things calmly, I have been called "Speedy Gonzales" since I was a child. It is as if time were not enough, mainly when I am working.

I am able to do what three people can do. My wife and I run a shop where 4 people used to work. My job makes me more and more nervous and I have to go faster and faster ... but on Sundays I forget all my responsibilities and go fishing. I love fishing because I feel calm. When I am in the water I can wait hours without catching a fish and I relax, but when I am out of there I cannot wait, even when I am in the street waiting at traffic-lights, especially if I have diarrhoea. It is even worse when I am in the middle of a crowd, it is a disaster, the more the people the stronger my disease, I feel faint.

I investigate:

"I have been having problems of dizziness since I was a child, I couldn't even go onto the slide! My legs shake and cannot bear me ... if I go onto a bridge or to the top of a tower it is a disaster, I could wet myself

[Translator note: wet is not intended as urinate, but as defecate].

He added spontaneously:

"All my problems with diarrhoea have worsened since I got to know I suffered of Paget disease. I think I will not have a good life anymore and I would like to spend the rest of my life in a better way".

His wife added that Oreste was on edge for any minimum matter, but most agitating was to know he has got an appointment.

Oreste highlighted:

"Years ago I used going fishing with some friends of mine, but I have not done it ever since because I always had to wait for them. Although it is Sunday morning ... if an appointment has been fixed, then it has to be respected, otherwise I get nervous and prefer to go away. I cannot wait ... otherwise I'd spoil my whole day"

Enquired on his child diseases, Oreste reminded all exanthemata diseases, parotitis accepted. Moreover he told me that at the age of four he was operated on tonsillectomy and adenoidectomy, I could not find out whether this was because of any particular problem. At the age of 27 Oreste was urgently operated on appendicectomy, which, according to his version "Was rapidly evolving into peritonitis".

Regarding his diet, the patient asserts having a real passion for sweets and any sort of citrus fruit, especially grape fruit and citron, of which he has been greedy since he was a child.

I prescribed ARGENTUM NITRICUM 200 CH.

10 days later Oreste called me showing strong aggravation of movements, up to 7-8-a-day, which barely allowed Oreste "to reach the lavatory".

I prescribed a placebo and three days after the situation had normalised.

After a month Oreste claimed pain in his arms and wrists that, according to his own words reminded him of first symptoms of the disease. Oreste was quite worried and the prescription of a placebo did not work out. I advised him of taking the 200 and in around a week the situation improved and pain disappeared.

After a few months, at Oreste's request, I met him and the patient said spontaneously:

"Diarrhoea has practically disappeared and the same for my hurry of going to the lavatory, I manage to go to the lavatory only once or twice a day, I feel free since I do not have diarrhoea any more and my stool is solid. My appetite has increased and I put on 4 kilos.

Till 10 days ago I was also feeling very calm, excepted while working. Now I feel as if there was too much to do. I am thinking of selling my shop and go back working as an employee, also because I am very easy to please and am content with what I have ... I have some money and would like to enjoy my life without all those responsibilities"

He added:

"Vertigoes have almost disappeared, although I am in the middle of a crowd ... And I managed to visit some friends who live at the eighth floor, I had always refused to visit them"

I enquired on the pains in his back:

"They worsened. In the past I almost did not feel any pain, now I feel a fastidious load on my back. But I feel better when my wife gives me a massage, above all if she is powerful while giving it to me. I wish somebody stretched my back, as if they used to do during tortures. My back burns. I feel much better when I lie in the sun"

He went on spontaneously:

"I have a strong desire of eating sweets, but I cannot eat citrus fruit anymore. I used to be very greedy of citrus fruit in the past, I almost feel sick if I only think of eating a citron. I used to get them directly from Sicily and Israel, since I was very greedy"

I prescribed him a dose of ARGENTUM NITRICUM 10M.

Almost three months later Oreste called me and said he was feeling much better: he did not claim any back aches and very first symptoms had disappeared "the agitation excepted" which, according to his words, showed up only at work: "I made up my mind of selling my shop; I think my work is ruining me. I am a calm man now ... but there is still something that does not allow me being serene. It is not because of money, but when I have to work I cannot go slowly"

Despite the subjective improvement of the disease, the laboratory exams highlighted a progressive advancement of the pathology, which was not accompanied by any characteristic symptom of Paget disease.

Alkaline phosphatasys and[1] hydroxiprolynuria were slowly rising progressively. Moreover, in my opinion Oreste had not really improved, I had the impression he was feeling more taken care of and that he was satisfied with the improvement of some of the symptoms, diarrhoea above all. The decision of leaving his business appeared to me as being a sort of escape, and at the same time the realisation of his dream of spending his last days of life as a *healthy person*. I got the right impression. In a separate interview his wife revealed me that Oreste was absolutely sure he would end sitting on a wheel chair and that anyway it would not be possible doing anything to cure his pathology, even to attenuate it.

I managed to convince the patient not to submit himself to (technetium bone) scintigraphy and the radiological state confirmed the alteration of trabecolar architecture of some of the vertebrae and of both the humeri.

Three months later Oreste decided to sell the shop, but after the new owner request Oreste made up his mind to remain working in the shop as an employee and of being, in facts, the only responsible.

A few weeks ago, I met the patient after his request. For the first time he had come alone. The strong pain in his arms and at cervical and dorsal rhachis had reappeared. Oreste claimed that all his pains improved with physical activities, especially in the open air. For this reason he started going jogging regularly with his wife.

He reported spontaneously:

"From a month I have gone back to the starting situation.

My father died and I started working harder and harder, now I am working up to 12 hours a day.

I have movements many times a day and often it is only mucus.

My sense of uneasiness while staying in a crowd has disappeared, and I do not have to run to the lavatory ... but I still need to go many times a day. Vertigoes have reappeared"

---

[1] N.d.t. "nel testo in italiano 'a'"

After a long silence Oreste lowered his eyes and said:

"I fancy making love only when I am on holiday, at home I feel too tired and sad to make it. Even though my wife keeps on insisting, I do not want to have any children because we would not have the time ... all that work I have to do"

I asked for more details, but I did not receive any reply.

Meanwhile his wife had become my patient, but she had always preferred coming alone. During our consultations the woman told me more than once that her husband refused decisively to face any argument regarding children. Before getting married Oreste asked her to promise that they would not even talk about the matter until they would reach a concrete economic steadiness. It had always been a taboo topic, even after a few years of marriage when they had reached a certain steadiness.

I collected information on the pain in his back:

"I usually feel a sense of heaviness and of formication. But when these feelings get stronger they become cramps, as if I my arms were pulled and I wish they could be pulled stronger to make my pain vanish, if I could I would hang by means of my arms and would put weights of 100 kilos on my feet.

I started eating sweets, but oranges and citrons make me sick"

I still prescribed him ARGENTUM NITRICUM but I did not observe any improvement. I am caparbious so I insisted, being convinced it were matter of power of the remedy, I tried with different potencies, but in the two following months the situation was still the same and Oreste started giving up hope.

Check ups showed that osteolisys had not aggravated further, but figures were always alarming. Without telling the doctors who were following him, the patient had not been taking any medicine.

After almost two months Oreste's fingers and wrists showed an exfoliate dermatitis, which caused great itching. His fingers were swollen and very irritated. Oreste said with peremptory tone:

"I will not go on with homeopathic therapy unless I see satisfying results soon".

I asked Oreste to see me again and the only new data, which had not been revealed until that moment, was a fastidious buzzing in his left ear. Oreste had had it for a very long time, but since his father death, it had become even more insistent:

"It is like a ring reminding me of my father ... he is there and the only thing I can do to forget him is to work, but now I am getting tired and I cannot bear this anymore.

Vertigoes are worsening and I cannot even screw a bulb in a lamp without feeling dizzy..."

Oreste also communicated me that his strong desire for sweets was now unbearable.

I reperorise the following symptoms:
1 - MIND - RESTLESSNESS - working, while
2 - VERTIGO - HIGH - places
3 - GENERALS - FOOD and DRINKS - sweets - desire
4 - MIND - INDUSTRIOUS, mania for work
5 - EAR - NOISES in - ringing
6 - EXTREMITIES - DISCOLORATION - Fingers - redness
7 - EXTREMITIES - ERUPTIONS - Fingers - scabs
8 - EXTREMITIES - ITCHING - Hand
9 - EXTREMITIES - ITCHING - Fingers
10 - EXTREMITIES - SWELLING - Fingers

The repertorisation highlighted a possibility for CITRUS VULGARIS.

While studying the remedy I found some of the symptoms also occurring in Oreste's case: loathing for oranges, pulling limb ache, wrists and arms cramps, want of open spaces. The MIND symptoms are those, which most attracted my attention: almost all of them are referred to agitation, very neat on work and to the need of operating in a zealous way.

The repertory does not show any symptom related to vertigo, while the *Allen* reports a form of frontal cefalgea accompanied by vertigoes. In *Allen* text only "osteolisys" symptoms are related to teeth that decay easily and as easily they are lost.

Unfortunately it was difficult for me to find the remedy in a short time, but I managed to get the mother tincture so I prepared a 6CH, which I asked him to take 3 times a day. Two days later the eruption was extended to the whole arms and was accompanied by a fastidious itching, "insomnia occurring with a sense of agitation" made its appearance, but back pains were progressively relieving.

A week later Oreste said he was feeling "different and strange" and after two weeks the patient admitted he had never felt so good before.

Meanwhile I managed to find a 30CH, but I still delayed to give it to the patient, since I wanted to wait for the evolution of the case.

After almost two months Oreste went back to the specialised medical centre where he was officially cured to be submitted to a routine check up: the laboratory exams had strongly improved. Eventually Oreste confessed that he had been following a homeopathic therapy. The doctors from the medical centre phoned me in order to know what I had given the patient.

For six months Oreste would not show any other symptom, meanwhile he changed his work and with his wife took over a newsagent kiosk. For the first time in his life Oreste has took up a job where he has to be sitting for a long time, almost immobile.

Occasionally he suffers of a pain in his cervical rhachis that disappears after a treatment of few drops of CITRUS VULGARIS 30CH.

After a few months Oreste got ill for a strong influence, having 40°C temperature, accompanied by diffused pains. The symptomatology was solved in a few hours with some drops of the remedy diluted in some water.

Eight years later Oreste has been considered as completely recovered by the doctors following his case at the specialised medical centre.

In this period of time I have occasionally prescribed him the remedy for banal episodes of headache and Oreste has always recovered in a few hours.

At the moment Oreste and his wife are the parents of a couple of twins and have moved to the hillside where they run a newsagent-kiosk.

Citrus vulgaris is very restless and has a strong tendency to overwork. In Citrus vulgaris and Citrus limonum there is always the feeling everything is too much, I have never done enough. It might look like Argentum nitricum, also diarrhoea, and anticipation.

Strong feeling of I am not strong enough to stand this responsibility.

In the noble metals we have the problem to handle the high expectations. Citrus and other Rutaceae are workaholics, but it is difficult to take responsibility.

Oreste did not want children, because it would have been too much for him.

The loss of the father is difficult to handle. Father in the sense of a myth.

They have to follow the will of that strict father, who is never satisfied with what they are doing.

In the **noble metals** we always find adored persons whose way has to be followed or overrated with the feeling I cannot. In Citrus it is never enough, but the grandiosity of the noble metals is lacking.

The difference with **Argentum** is that in Argentum you see a person who is taking responsibility and trying to do something big. In Citrus they do less, they would like to do something big, but they cannot. It is not so important what goal to reach, but it is important to work.

Diarrhoea is very common in Citrus. Orange juice can cause destruction of the bones and the enamel of the teeth.

CUPRUM METALLICUM

Scientific Latin Name: Cuprum metallicum

Traditional Names:

English: copper

German: Kupfer

Etymology

The name "copper" is derived from the Latin term *"cuprum"*, which itself comes from the term *"as cyprium"*, ore from the island of Cyprus (Greek: *Kypros*).

Classification

Minerals; inorganic; precious metals; copper-group;

The element copper:

Chemical symbol: Cu

Atomic mass: 63.546

Atomic number: 29

Density: 8960 kg m^{-3}

Melting point: 1357 K

Boiling point: 2840 K

Copper is positioned in the periodic table in group 1b, the same as the precious metals silver and gold, and in the 4th period between nickel and zinc. In this period we also find the elements potassium, calcium, germanium and arsenic (a-group elements), as well as the b-group elements chromium, manganum, iron and cobalt.

Keywords

Precious metal

Used Parts

Trituration of the metal

Description of the Substance

Copper is a shiny reddish soft malleable and extremely ductile metal, which conducts heat and electrical current very well (second only to silver, the third best conductor being gold). Copper vapour shines with a bluish-green light. It forms valuable alloys with many metals, e.g. bronze with tin and brass with zinc. In compounds it can have a valence of +1 or +2; the bivalent salts are blue or green, the monovalent ones colourless. In humid air copper acquires a layer of basic copper carbonate (patina), with solutions containing acetic acid (also with fruits in copper vessels) it forms a basic copper acetate (verdigris). The latter is poisonous and was used in former times in painting as a pigment (Spanish green, in German called "Gruenspan"). The surface of the metal appears brownish-red, but when looking through a fine layer of the metal it appears blue green. Its salt solutions display hews of blue green, green and violet, as mentioned already. In its ores it shows its colourfulness as well: golden in copper pyrite ($CuFeS2$), green in malachite and olivenite, blue in azurite, violet blue in cove line, and in the coloured copper pyrite (chalcopyrite) it displays all the colours of the rainbow. Copper (II)- chloride is used in fireworks due to the green colour of its flame.

Deposits:

Copper is found in the free metallic state in nature, especially in basaltic lava. The largest known deposit of copper is found in the Andean mountains in Chile, due to volcanic activity. Concerning the distribution of copper over the earth the most deposits are found in the western continents, a medium amount in the middle continents and very few in the eastern continents. America possesses about 35% of the earth's copper deposits, Europe 11%, Africa 18% and Australia 1%. The greatest amount of copper is found around the Pacific.

The most important copper ores are sulphur compounds, which are mainly found at great depths, in the so-called basic molten rocks, which are poor in quartz. It is not frequently found within the silicon-containing rocks of the earth's surface (pyrites and granite) – similar to the fact that silicic acid in animal organisms also moves to the surface (hair, skin, sense organs), whereas copper remains predominantly deeper under the surface, e.g. as a component of the blood of molluscs. The most common copper ore is copper *pyrite* (chalcopyrite), a copper-iron-sulphide. Other iron –copper compounds contain silver, gold, mercury, lead, tin, arsenic or antimony. When these ores come to the oxygen-rich surface, the iron contained starts to rust, leaving iron-free *coppersulfide,* e.g. *copper-pyrite.* The most stable form resulting from all the metamorphoses of copper is the basic copper carbonate, emerald green *malachite*, which forms due to the influence of carbonic acid and water. So copper moves out of the sphere of sulfur into the sphere of oxygen and carbonic acid. Copper is found in low concentration all over the planet, being equivalent to the 4th decimal power.

Traditional use

Copper was discovered and first used during the Neolithic period, or New Stone Age. This is believed to have been about 8000 BC.The native copper is the material that humans employed as a substitute for stone. Its use for tools, implements, weapons and artwork dates at least from 4000 BC in Chaldea. In Egypt the first devices made out of copper date back to the years 3900 to 3600 BC. From 3100 BC on the Bronze Age follows, during which man discovered that copper alloys using tin or zinc were both more durable and easier to work with. Then after another Copper Age the Main Bronze Age is dated starting around 2100 BC. In the Middle Ages the copper and slate mines of Mansfeld supplied the whole European continent for centuries with the metal. People came into contact with copper daily by using door handles, kettles, coins and implements of art and daily use. The more iron took its place, the more copper moved back into the sphere of arts.

This situation changed dramatically the moment the nature of electricity and magnetism was discovered. Copper, which was originally smelted out of its ores using the fire process, could now produce itself in a pure form through electricity – by means of copper electrodes through electrolysis. As copper has been assigned since ancient times to the goddess Venus, to femininity, in contrast to iron, which was assigned to Mars, the god of war and the male principle, one could continue this idea, saying copper has emancipated itself with the help of electricity. It is difficult to imagine the world without the use of electromagnetism. Generators display an interaction between iron and copper, in order to bring electricity into the world for the production of heat, light, and kinetic energy and not least as a prerequisite for data transfer (copper cables, electromagnetic radio waves, etc.).

Copper makes a melodious sound and is used in the production of wind and percussion instruments. The basic copper acetate (verdigris) is poisonous and was used in former times in painting as a pigment (Spanish green).

Myths, Legends, Ritual Use

According to Greek mythology, the goddess Aphrodite (in Roman mythology Venus) rose from foaming waves out of a seashell (that is, a mollusc whose haemoglobin contains copper) off the coast of Cyprus. The element copper, the day of the week Friday, (in German and English named after the goddess Freya, in Italian venerdi, the day of Venus) and the planet Venus are all ascribed to this goddess.

The Chaldean Order:

The Chaldeans put the planets known at that time (and visible with the naked eye) including the sun and the moon and with them the corresponding metals and gods in a certain order, which points to a remarkable knowledge of the cosmic and physical correlations and which our modern names and order of the days of the week are based on.

Some examples:

If we put the seven planet-metals in a line according to their *atomic mass*, the following order results:

Fe - Cu - Ag - Sn - Au - Hg - Pb corresponding to

Mars - Venus - Moon - Jupiter - Sun - Mercury - Saturn.

If we put these metals in a circular order in the form of a heptagon, the resulting correlations are interesting:

Gold takes a special position on top in the middle, while the other metals face each other in pairs, according to their combined occurrence in nature and their parallel or counter effects within the organism.

If we draw an **acute-àngled seven-pointed star** into a circle, the resulting order of the planets shows their distances from the earth, beginning with the most distant, Saturn, and ending with the nearest, the moon. If we draw an **obtuse-angled seven-pointed star**, a *temporal* order of world events results instead of a spatial order. The order of the days of the week brings into consciousness our seven-based rhythm.

Sun – Sunday – gold
Moon – Monday – (lunedi) – silver
Mars – Tuesday (Ziu = Germanic god of war) – (martedi) – iron
Mercury – Wednesday (Wotan = Germanic equivalent of Mercury) – (merco-ledi) - quicksilver
Jupiter – Thursday (Germanic god Donar or Thor) – (giovedi) – tin
Venus – Friday (Germanic goddess Freyja, Freia) – (venerdi)- copper
Saturn – Saturday – lead (plumbum –guardian of the threshold)

The more distant planets Neptune, Uranus and Pluto cannot be seen by the naked eye, they are beyond human range. Until now, the human body has not been able to deal with radioactive elements like neptunium, uranium and plutonium Lead as the guardian of the threshold_protects us; there is the possibility of black magic on the one hand and spirituality on the other hand - destruction or the next evolutionary step, when we can handle these forces.

There are many other correlations concerning this order of the planets, e.g. the intervals of tones in music, the electric resistance of metals, the order of the chakras, etc.

Toxicology, Pharmacy, Medicine

Certain copper compounds can be very poisonous for lower forms of plants and animals (copper coins put into an aquarium prevent its infestation with algae) and are therefore used as pesticides. Higher developed organisms are less sensitive; for many plants and animals copper is an essential trace element (serving as a component of the blood of molluscs, squids and crustaceans – hemocya-nine; mint-balm contains a lot of copper). Certain birds (such as turakos) pro-duce the red, blue, green and violet hues of their feathers with the help of cop-per. All organisms, which use copper as the central atom of the porphyrine for respiration, have in common that their skeleton has been transferred to the sur-face in the form of a protecting layer (forms such as seashells and snail shells), that their body temperature is dependant on the surroundings (cold-blooded animals), and that they lack a voice. The development of a voice is connected to the breathing of air; land-dwelling molluscs are still close to the watery element and also use hem cyanine as their blood pigment.

In the human organism, copper is found in *Warburg's respiration enzyme* (cyto-chromoxidase), in the human serum it is contained in another oxidase, the func-tion of which is not yet understood. Copper is necessary for the oxidation and absorption of vitamin C during digestion. Copper also acts as a catalyst in the formation of haemoglobin. In human erythrocytes a blue copper-containing protein is found *(hemocupreine),* which probably has an influence on the activ-ity of histamine. Copper as an essential trace element is necessary for erythro-poesis (daily requirement 2 mg). The level of copper in the serum (normally 12 – 24 μmol/l = 70 – 150μg/dl) is higher in cases of anaemia due to iron defi-ciency, in tumours, infections, M. Basedow and during pregnancy. The liver is particularly rich in copper. Copper seems to have a certain kind of protecting effect against cholera; the disease nearly never affected copper workers.

A continuous influx of small amounts of copper salts causes numerous symp-toms (as known from homoeopathic provings): depression, fear of death, ver-tigo and disturbances in body temperature, with coldness pouring into the whole body. Malfunctions of the respiratory, digestive and urinary tracts are known with a tendency to produce cramps. Paracelsus tried to cure mental diseases, epilepsy, lung diseases and syphilis with copper. Whooping cough, intestinal parasites, venous congestion and varicose veins have been treated with the metal as well.

M. Wilson, hepatolenticular degeneration, is caused by a hereditary malfunction in the metabolism of copper and the production of caeruloplasmine. (*Caerulo-plasmine* is a copper transporting protein; normally 95% of the copper in the serum is bound to it.) Symptoms include extra pyramidal syndrome with hyperkinesias, flapping tremor and myoklonia, disturbance of affectivity and memory, psychosis, possible mental degeneration in the last stage and also hepatosplenomegalia. The *Kayser-Fleischer-corneal ring,* an olive-green ring in the peripheral descemet membrane, is path gnomonic. Therapy: potassium sulphide, which prevents the incorporation, and D- penicillamine, which enhances the elimination of copper.

Overall, it may be said that copper, which is a component of the blood pigment in lower animals, leaves this task to iron in human beings, but is still necessary for the production of haemoglobin allowing for the integration of iron into the haemoglobin and for cellular respiration. W*arm* blood develops and the breathing of air, which allows for the development of the voice, and the calcium is transferred to the centre and formed into an inner skeleton. Copper is predominantly assigned to the metabolic, liver and venous regions and to the unformed aspects, and according to the anthroposophic view it serves to prepare the higher self-organisation.

Discussion of Cuprum Themes

Spasmodic tendency

Convulsions, spasms, cramps, twitching, jerking – expressed in various organs: Nerves, cerebrospinal axis, muscles of digestive and respiratory tract, skeletal muscles. In any protoplasma the most basic reaction is the retraction after an external stimulus. It is the primary defence mechanism against any external influence ranging from a simple touch to a threatening attack.

We can find cramps on the physical as well as on the emotional level, mostly in form of paroxysms. Convulsions on the physical level may start in the fingers and toes, from the periphery inward. We can find epileptic attacks, leading to unconsciousness and even coma. The causation might be a suppression of skin diseases, foot sweat and various discharges, emotions, anger, overtaxing, loss of sleep or even touch. There are symptoms like spasmodic cough or respiratory affections with short periods in which breathing stops. The patients might appear as if they were dead with blueness and coldness of the surface. We also can find behavioural problems: striking, shrieking, biting, spitting, temper tantrums, imitating and making ridiculous gestures and grimaces, playing the jolly joker.

Their sense of humour might be very offending. On the emotional level these patients are serious, self –critical and cramped inside as well. This spasmodic reaction on the emotional level is their answer to their

Feeling of being in a vulnerable position and being threatened by an external attack

They always have to be alert due to their fear of doing things wrong, making mistakes. They stay exactly within the rules and want others do the same. They will report on another who violates the rules.

They are generally ambitious and show perseverance and fanaticism, dislike being looked at or touched. They feel easily criticized, insulted and even persecuted and then might get angry, kick, punch, scream and break things.

Their idea of vulnerability and their fear of making mistakes leads to the fear of being approached, pursued by the police and the delusion that they are about to be arrested. They have an aversion to company and strangers, cannot bear anyone near them. Their vulnerability shows itself in a feeling of being attacked personally –

DD.: *Aurum* - *my* whole country is attacked, because I am the king.

DD. between the vulnerability of the *compositae* and the precious metals:

The compositae are much more vulnerable, they don't want to be touched because of their fear of being injured, in the precious metals (esp. *Aurum, Argentum, Platina*) this is because of a feeling of superiority. The compositae are much more concerned with the integrity of their own body. Many compositae like arnica, bellis perennis, erigeron, and calendula are used as vulnerary plants. They are able to push the vital force to reconstruct as soon as possible. These persons are often in a position of command, but never at the top of the hierarchy, often they are people who are executing orders. This is similar to *Cuprum* (as will be explained in the following), whereas *Ferrum* is more in the direction of being a good soldier.

One possibility of compensation in cuprum is that they try to control everything in a rigid way. They must always stretch themselves to meet everyone's wishes. If you have cramps in your calves, you will walk on your toes. (Linda Johnston). They are fastidious, conscientious and get angry if others don't obey the rules as they do.

Another possible compensation is to become a general oneself. (*Delusion he is a general, a great person, an officer*). He takes an aura of command and becomes dictatorial. Deep within he feels that he never will be able to reach a position of the leader or the king like *aurum.* He believes, that people will think he is ordinary, (Del. selling vegetables, repairing old chairs) so he tries to hide this by giving himself an air of importance.

In the decompensated state we can find a fear of losing position or command in *Aurum*, whereas in the case of *Cuprum, Arnica* or *Bellis perennis* you do not see this. Their main problem is that they are not as strong as they were before, people can see how weak they are.

Concerning the physical body, the *Compositae* are more affecting the liver and muscles, in the precious metals there are problems in the eyes, the gonads, the circulation and the heart. They have much more to do with the central system. *Cuprum, Argentum and Aurum* can be used as disinfectants; they are antibacterial. We don't have this kind of situation in the same way for the *compositae.* Even if *Calendula* is a very good antibacterial, it is much more in the direction of reconstruction, building the previous order.

Superiority

Cuprum is in the middle of the precious metals and the compositae concerning dignity and honour. He can behave haughty, but he also can have a fear of falling and of high places in a more decompensated state. He is the chief of the army of aurum. Cuprum is always at the service of somebody else. So in old age, when cuprum becomes decompensated, he is more able to accept the idea of losing his power. He is able to recognise that he reached something, and he is content enough of what he did. Usually the peak they have to reach is not as high as in aurum, so it is sufficient for them to be continuously honoured and esteemed. They have less problems in having a friendly relationship with others, and they are able to perceive at the end of their life they could be something humble, and remembering life as is was before. Very often you can find the classic picture of an old general that is always telling stories of what he did when he was young, of beautiful battles, etc.
DD.: *Aurum* wants to continue his empire when he is old.

Integration of/ Problems with the Male/Female Side:

Cuprum is the Venus that has transformed to a general. The feminine side is not so well integrated.

In cuprum and the precious metals like aurum, platina, etc. we often can find an over demanding father. But in cuprum this father loses his power at a certain moment and it is as if cuprum has to do what his father could not do. DD.: *Aurum has* a father who is really strong and he must make it even better.

Summary Cuprum themes

Spasmodic tendency

Feeling of being in a vulnerable position and being threatened by an external attack

Superiority

Integration of/ Problems with the male/female side

The Original Proving

Was done by Samuel Hahnemann.

Bibliography

Sieben Metalle - Wilhelm Pelikan (Philosophisch-Antroposophischer Verlag Goetheanum)

Schüler - Duden Die Chemie (Dudenverlag Mannheim/Leipzig/Wien/Zürich)

Duden Das Herkunftswörterbuch (Bibliographisches Institut Mannheim / Wien / Zürich)

Klinisches Wörterbuch - Pschyrembel 257. Auflage (De Gruyter)

Internet: Encyclopedia Britannica

and in the "homoeopathy-part": seminar-notes of Linda Johnston and Nick Churchill.

ACIDS

Substance:

Chemically, acids are either proton donators, that is, they are capable of dissociating into hydrogen ions (protons) and anions when dissolved in water, or they are hydroxide acceptors, meaning they are able to bind the hydroxide ions (OH-ions) of the water solution, so that relatively more protons are left in the solution.

Weak acids only dissociate to a low degree.

The pH-value is a measure of the acidic or basic (alkaline) nature of a solution. The concentration of the hydrogen ion (H+) activity in a solution determines the pH.

There are organic and inorganic acids, organic acids dissociate less than inorganic.

There is a close relationship to metals. Acids affect some metals like vanadium, copper, and zinc. "Königswasser" (Aqua regia, Kings Water) (HCL + Acidum salicylicum) even dissolves gold. Inorganic acids are stronger acids and more destructive than organic acids.

General themes of acids

Losing someone or something

Weakness
Complaining silently
Deep suffering
Cowardice
Greediness
Cupidity

Loss of stability and structure (dissolving)

Injuries

Concentration difficulty
Chilliness

Cold destructive environment

Bad relationship with mother, poisonous intake since beginning, not only bad feeding but acid feeding. Hungry, but gets poison, therefore they are so sensitive to real loss. It is a disaster when they lose the person they once managed to trust.

Self destruction

Consuming themselves for others
Poor persons with a lot of problems
Difficulty to communicate
Strong sense of duty
Depression

Corrosion of skin and mucosa

Ulcers
Constriction
Burning, stitching pains
Cramps
Paralysing

Differences between *organic and inorganic acids*:

Inorganic: mental state is stronger
             Burning, pressing pain
Organic: deeply suffering without expressing a lot
             Loss of fluids
             Less destructive
             More sore pain

209

MURIATICUM ACIDUM

Description

Chlorum Cl 2 is a yellow-green gas with stinging odour, hygroscopic and not inflammable. Its melting point is minus 102,0°C, its boiling point minus 34,1°C. It reacts easily and with hydrogen it builds a mixture of gases that react with each other under explosion. **"Chlorknallgas"**: H2 + Cl2 ---> 2 HCl. This Chlorhydrogen is a colourless gas with stinging odour, dissolves itself easily in water whereby it gives a proton to the water molecule and so H3O+ arises.

The gases melting point is minus 113°C, its boiling point minus 85°C. The solution in water contains 37% HCl and is a strong mineral acid, which is also called vaporizing hydrochloric acid. It dissolves continuously the gas into the air.

A mixture of HCL and HNO3 is called **kings water**, because it can dissolve gold. Being an important reactive in chemical labour the acid reacts with NH3 (ammonia) to NH4Cl (chloride of ammonium).

With not precious metals it easily forms salts, always building chlorides, like
Ferrum + HCl ---> FeCl + hydrogen
Magnesium + HCL ---> MgCl + hydrogen
Sodium + HCl ---> NaCl + hydrogen

Iron rusts easily under the influence of HCl. Copper is not touched by HCl, but copper oxide is.

With Calcarea (CaCO3) there is a reaction that evolves CO2, if you put HCl on a Calcarea stone it will foam. So one can distinguish it from a Silicea containing stone, which will not foam.

Sources
Hydrochloric gas originates from a reaction of chlorum with hydrogen. This reaction can under the influence of light be an explosion.

In the laboratory the gas can rise from a reaction of sodium chloride and sulphuric acid (first described by the pharmacist and chemist Rudolph Glauber in the 17th century). From this process derives the German name Salzsäure, which means acid, made of salt.

Today hydrochloric acid is produced in organic chemistry processes, when adding chlorum to organic substances like the production of PVC, where HCl is a side   product.

Ethan + Chlor --------> Dichlorethan --------> Vinylchlorid + Hydrochloric acid

$H_2C=CH_2 + Cl_2$ --------> ClH_2C-CH_2Cl --------> $H_2C=CHCl + HCl$

Since the HCl is an important factor of pollution and on the other hand a potential good, a recycling processes of industrial gases is just being developed to optimise the washing of gases deriving from refuse incineration plants to gain a pure hydrochloric acid that can be used and sold again.

HCl and pollution

Hydrochloric acid plays an important role for the destruction of ozone in the stratosphere. It derives mainly from FCKW that are emitted by a huge industry using chlorum as a main substance for many products. In the stratosphere they are photo chemically deconstructed and release ozone-diminishing radicals. They transform odd oxygen's (O and O3) into even ones (O2) and can only leave the stratosphere by sinking down and being washed out and transforming to sour rain that damages the flora and buildings.

A natural source of ozone destructing radicals is emissions of volcanoes, where HCl and H2SO4 reach the stratosphere and stay there for 12 to 18 months. During this period a decrease of ozone can be proved.

(translated   and   shortened   version   from: pluslucis.univie.ac.at/FBA/FBA99/Sonnweber)

Traditional and nowadays use

Neutralisation of CaCO3 in industry.

Formerly used to a much smaller extent for removing rests of Calcarea from ceramics.

Regulation of pH and removal of Calcarea in swimming pools.

For regeneration of kations exchange machines, which together with anion exchange machines, are needed to produce water purer than distilled

Analysis in hydrolytic chemistry, e.g. splitting up proteins to prove the composition of foods.

Food addition and poison
It is added to dog food to make it spicier due to chlorpropanoles that arise during the process, but then the food becomes cancerous.
Food addition substance E 507 is HCl. They use it mainly for producing sugar out of starch of maize. During this process chlorated sterines and chlorpropanoles arise which were used as poison for rats.

First chemical weapon that was used worked with phosgene, which releases HCl when touching mucous membranes and brings on internal corrosion. Death arises from stoppage of respiratory function after several hours.

Artistic use: Dutch bath (C. Fleck)
For artistic etching of copper, zinc and brass the use of the Dutch bath is recommended. It contains water, HCl and KCl.

Physiology

Hydrochloric acid is contained in the stomach in a concentration of 0,3%. It is needed for digestion enzyme Carboanhydrase they produce carbonic acid out of water and carbodioxide. The dissociating H+ is actively transported into the lumen together with an equal number of Cl-. The blood leaving the stomach contains more HCO3- and has a much higher pH then before (especially after meals). A mucous layer protects the stomach from self-digestion.

Toxicology

Skin:
Corrosion of the skin is very painful, reddened and swollen. With deeper corrosions all layers of the skin and deeper issues can be affected, though there is a self-limited progredience because of the precipitation of the proteins that form an impermeable layer to the acid.

Eyes:

By injuries or attacks the acid can be sprinkled into the eyes.

There are immediate heavy pains when the cornea is injured. In cases that remain on the surface the cornea stays clear and transparent, with deeper lesions there is a milky obscuration and loss of vision.

Mouth, pharynx and oesophagus:

Erroneous ingestion can irritate the mucous membranes but can also lead to necrosis and ulceration, e.g. of the stomach. The event is very painful, there is an increased salivation, the mucous membranes of the mouth and digestive tract are dry, bleeding, cracked and deeply ulcerated. Later scars are formed and can lead to strictures and hindrances of passage.

There is increased incidence of malign tumours in these regions after many years.

Respiratory tract:

The acute injury by inhaling Chlorgas appears as corrosion mainly caused by chloric acid. The mucus membranes of mouth, pharynx, and larynx down to the lungs can be damaged. We find hoarseness, cough and burning pain during respiration. Deep inhalation leads to oedema of lungs and pneumonia.

Blood:

This acid has an elective affinity for the blood, producing a septic condition similar to that found in low fevers with high temperature and great prostration, restlessness.

Violent haemorrhages (e.g. in brain – petechial and perivascular haemorrhage without reaction)
Decomposition of blood- bluish tongue, piles, ulcers.

Muscles:

are affected and exhausted, especially of heart (angina pectoris), of bladder, anus, tongue etc., causing paresis. Pulsations in single parts.

Homeopathy

The main action of potentized Hydrochloric Acid is on typhoid conditions, especially those of a septic kind, in which the patient slides down in the bed owing to great weakness, the lower jaw hangs down, and the tongue is dry, leathery and shrivelled, maybe with deep ulceration, bluish-red edges of aphthous ulcers; there is a dirty coating on the teeth, the breath is offensive, and there is a swelling of the gums and local lymphatic nodes. The uvula may also be swollen with ulceration and membranes, so that attempts to swallow give rise to spasms and attacks of choking, resulting in a state of extreme prostration, in which, without realizing it, the patient may pass urine, and urination may be accompanied by involuntary defecation (after radiotherapy).

In such serious typhoid conditions the pulse is frequently weak, small and rapid and misses every third beat (cf. Kali carb.). Lying on the right side, before midnight and in damp weather, markedly aggravates the patient whereas lying on the left side ameliorates.

There is a typical aversion to meat with periodically ravenous hunger and continual craving for drinks, with abdominal rumbling owing to fermentation of food. Rectal problems are also typical, on the one hand characterized by involuntary defecation on urination, and on the other hand by haemorrhoids, which are so sensitive to touch, that even the use of toilet paper is painful. Pruritus ani may occur, with anal prolapse on urination.

Haemorrhoids in pregnancy are also characteristic, bluish in colour, hot and with violent sticking pains.

In spite of incontinence of urine, the patient must wait a long time for the urine to arrive, accompanied by simultaneous involuntary defecation. Impotence may also be present in men.

There are rheumatic cutting and drawing pains in the limbs, better for movement (cf. Rhus tox.) and worse at rest. Toothache in incipient caries is much worse from cold drinks.

The patient is easily provoked, more irritable than usual, with a tendency to anger, or also to gloom and melancholy with general apathy and discontent.

The characteristic skin symptoms of Muriatic Acid include burning with itching in a wide variety of places, especially the scrotum, barely relieved by scratching and giving rise to the eruption of vesicles and the formation of scabs with small painful nodules and pustules and consequent suppuration with burning and itching. Ulcers may form, with offensive discharge and looking like burns, especially on the lower leg. There is a typical eczema of the hand.

A characteristic of Muriatic Acid is also the general sensitivity to the slightest touch, especially in haemorrhoids and on the genitalia.

Muriaticum acidum themes

DD to other *syphilitic remedies* :completely devoted to someone else.

Submissive – to do everything to please others. Come from a poor environment, lot of needs, but not able to receive anything he needs. Consume themselves to maintain one good relationship. Sacrifice themselves, always in the periphery and help his environment to work. "I do not deserve it, but I have to sacrifice myself to be allowed to stay here." Strong persons, never ask for anything, never recognized for what they are doing. Over helping, overdoing, not doing anything for himself. People can take advantage of them. Reproduce a similar situation as in their family and do not get anything back. And they feel they deserve this. Ph-ac and all strong acids arrive at a state of being worn out, not a matter of an objective stress, but more an emotional worn out, centred on a relationship.

Separation, loss, not be loved is breaking point for the acids.

Slaves who love their torturer.

Muriaticum: resentment, staying in bad experiences and feeling crashed by them after a time. Resignation. No egotism at all. (DD metals, Ammoniums, Digitalis)
Digitalis is dictatorial, does everything for others without being asked, but demands a lot in return.
Vexation.
Ammonium muriaticum – chemically two very different aspects. Ammonium: haughty, nasty people, want to be different (Palladium).
Staphisagria would be more active; there is more rage!

Muriaticum Acidum had difficulty to cope with other people, not so much haughty. After many years in their decompensated state, they may try to get back all they have given to the others. This greediness can be insisting and nasty, even aggressive. Intention to show the others how much they are suffering. Mostly no good relation with the doctor, little confidence. They come as seldom as possible. Never experienced confidence in the support of others.

Case 70-year-old lady

First consultation at the age of 61, owning a huge store in the centre of a village selling everything.

Terrible stomachache, helicobacter – treatment without effect. Took lots of medicines without result.

Attitude to consume a lot of medicines, even if intoxicated they do not stop (all acids).

Never could have kids, can stand on her feet because she has a lot of grudge, her main energy. Suffering because husband separated 20 years ago, but still lives in the same house.

" It is as if I was his servant. He was a Don Giovanni and I would have left him, but my mother forced me to stay with him so people would not talk about her. I am his slave without money. He has no culture, I thought him how to live and now I am sucked out.

Something going out of my stomach, feet and head. I am an empty sack that must continue to walk, because every day he comes home for lunch and for dinner."

Long list of all people who died in her family with very bad diseases and she gave them a lot of support. (There is more feeling of duty, not so much of a real sympathy).

"Since 20 years I have stained my underwear. Three curettages already, but all the remedies I am taking go directly into my urine, chemical trash that comes out of my kidney.

Continuous leucorrhoea, but also drops of urine, kind of violet stuff. I must take anti-depressive medication because my husband is a dirty stupid man.

The day I wanted to divorce I got pneumonia. My father told me, if you separate from this man it is like killing me." Cries.

"He gave me nothing, no money. He is older than me but still goes to the discotheque."

Ignatia made her dream again, but nothing else. "My mind was unblocked, but my husband said I am stealing his money "

Dream: " Field full of grass, all of a sudden I have to stop because there is a hole. Stop because of fear of falling down. Wake up because I am falling.

Or running down stairs, but then fall because there are no steps anymore".

"Most important thing was to have a child, but we could not, because my husband had a nephritis. But the dirt is not in my house, it is in my husbands."

Severe constipation, must remove stool with fingers.

Awful flatulence, swallowing lots of air.

Coldness, mainly in feet.

Cannot talk with anybody – too tired for deeper conversation.

"My soul is always forcing me to think about my past, but it is such an effort to think how I was yrs ago. To be nice takes away all my energy. Thinking of previous times is like opening a painful wound. I lost everything. I rent my store, and this person stole everything in my store.

I am considered a lady, but all that money is in the pocket of my husband. A bitter sting in my heart. The money is mine, and I have to ask him for money every week."

In his Muriaticum Acidum – cases Massimo has often seen much bitterness and resignation in the patient. In the decompensate state the greediness can be really insisting in trying to get something that is not possible. Coming from a bad environment they reproduce the same situation. After many years they sometimes try to get back all they have given with the intention to show to others how much they are suffering. There can be a lot of aggression. In one case Massimo prescribed *Sepia* first, because of the tremendous aversion towards the children.

SULPHURICUM ACIDUM

Description

Sulphuric acid, H_2SO_4, is a colourless viscous corrosive oily liquid, which has
    Melting Point: 10.3 degC
    Boiling Point: 338 degC

Formula weight 98.08

Specific gravity or density 1.94

Flash point none

Sulphuric Acidum is the strong acid produced by dissolving sulphur trioxide in water.

$SO3 + H2O ==> H2SO4$

It is a powerful protonating agent. It is also a moderately strong oxidizing agent.

Sulphuric acid is also a powerful dehydrating agent and is used to remove a molecule of water from many organic compounds.

In dilute solution, sulphuric acid is a strong dibasic acid forming two series of salts.

It is an important industrial chemical and it has many uses as a strong oxidizing agent and a powerful dehydrating agent.

Commercially sulphuric acid is available as a 96-98% solution of the acid in water.

The dehydration reactions of alcohols result in their conversion into an alkene, and involve the elimination of a molecule of water. Dehydration requires the presence of an acid and the application of heat.

What causes acid rain?

One of the main causes of acid rain is sulphur dioxide. Natural sources that emit this gas are volcanoes, sea spray, rotting vegetation and plankton. However, the burning of fossil fuels, such as coal and oil, are largely to be blamed for approximately half of the emissions of this gas in the world. When sulphur dioxide reaches the atmosphere, it oxidizes to first form a sulphate ion. It then becomes sulphuric acid as it joins with hydrogen atoms in the air and falls back down to earth. Oxidation occurs the most in clouds and especially in heavily polluted air where other compounds such as ammonia and ozone help to catalyse the reaction, converting more sulphur dioxide to sulphuric acid. However, not the entire sulphur dioxide is converted to sulphuric acid. In fact, a substantial amount can float up into the atmosphere, move over to another area and return to earth unconverted.

Nitric oxide and nitric dioxide are also components of acid rain. Its sources are mainly from power stations and exhaust fumes. Like sulphur dioxide, these nitrogen oxides rise into the atmosphere and are oxidized in clouds to form nitric acid. These reactions are also catalysed in heavily polluted clouds where iron, manganese, ammonia and hydrogen peroxide are present.

Physiology

The dilute acids act in the stomach chemically. Secretion is promoted by nitric acid, lessened by sulphuric acid; hydrochloric acid acts between the other two. They check the flow to mouths of ducts having an acid secretion; to those of alkaline secretion they promote flow (e.g., bile, pancreatic juice, etc.). The mineral acids check fermentation. Bowels are constipated by sulphuric, relaxed by nitric acid.

As these agents are synergistic to pepsin, they at first aid digestion; but if continued they lessen the production of gastric juice, and so impair digestion, Given before meals in small doses they will relieve excessive acidity of the stomach, by checking the production of the acid gastric juice.

Toxicology

The strong acids are escharotics, abstracting the water from the tissues, combining with the bases, destroying the protoplasm, and are very diffusible. Sulphuric carbonises (black); nitric tans (yellow)

Poisoning by mineral acids is treated by alkalis, as washing soda, soap-suds, etc., to neutralize the acid; after the stomach has been emptied cautiously, oil, albumen, or milk is given to protect the mucous membrane. Stimulants, opium and ammonia an applied intravenously, to combat the resulting depressed condition of the vital powers.

Traditional and nowadays use

Therapeutics:
The mineral acids are used in atonic dyspepsia, small doses of hydrochloric acid with pepsin, given after meals, except where there is acidity of the stomach.

Acidity —hydrochloric or phosphoric acids in small doses before meals.

Oxaluria —nitric or nitro-hydrochloric acid.

Lithaemia - nitric acid.

Diarrhoea—when profuse secretions, sulphuric acid with opium or with magnesium sulphate is found very serviceable. Fevers—especially typhoid, — hydrochloric acid is preferred.

Lead poisoning—sulphuric acid, to form the insoluble sulphate of lead.

Haemorrhoids—sulphuric acid; also for haemorrhage from lower bowel.

Haemorrhages—sulphuric acid is undoubtedly effective in uterine haemorrhage from fibroids, and in other haemorrhages at points distant from the stomach; also sometimes in haemorrhagica purpura.

Chronic hepatic disorders, —nitro-hydrochloric acid in all forms of liver affections due to malaria, internally, and locally as a bath.

Intermittent and remittent fevers, —nitric acid in full doses, is beneficial.

Aphonia of singers, —dilute nitric acid in 10-drop doses, has proved efficient.

Phthisis—aromatic sulphuric acid for the sweats.

Locally applied they are employed against:

Ulcers—fuming nitric acid as an escharotic, also in gangrene.

Haemorrhoids of the bleeding strawberry-pile kind—fuming nitric acid.

Diseased joints—Counter-irritation by Brodie's liniment, composed of sulphuric acid one-fourth and olive oil, three-fourths.

Uterine Diseases are often treated with fuming Nitric Acid, locally applied.

Sulphuricum acidum themes

Hurrying aimless

Impatience

Fruitless activity

Weakness of memory

Mistakes in talking

Flushes of heat

Haemorrhage, blood does not coagulate

Pressing pains

External pressure amel.

Burning pains

Homeopathy

Sulfuricum acidum as a homeopathic remedy is not so easy to understand. It is seldom prescribed, though being a big remedy. It can be very helpful to know the general themes of the acids. It is a
STRONG ACID, but there are not many mind symptoms in the repertory.
Injuries – only hint to self-destructiveness
Massimo's cases were always addicted out of a social situation. Like Heroin...
Ailments from injuries – common to persons with frequent injuries, awkwardness that drives towards situations where one can easily be injured.
Always leaking part that destroys the form in the acids. In Sulfuricum Acid this leaking part could be the injuries.

Sick person with greediness of being taken care for. Strategy similar to those of some **spiders:** Progressive, self-destructive diseases to give back what they received badly from their supporter. They remain in the family and suffer tremendously in front of them. Similar in Sulfuric Acid. Restlessness, hurry, dependent, capricious.

Sulphuricum Acidum's similarity to the **Sulphur** side: presenting himself as the hypothetical philosopher who produces strange metaphilosophical ideas, trying to give out the impression that he knows and you don't. It is not so easy to know what he knows. "Stillita"(Italy): holy people living on a tree or column, watching the world from upside.

Strong sense of anger, which is easy to perceive. Try to be supported in a peculiar way. Instead of doing something practical they do their best in a confused and unsuccessful way, fruitless activity, chaotic. No precise plan in what they are doing, give the impression to do more than they can. Feeling that it is not recognized what they are doing. Stay close to the family knowing everything better that the family should do, which house to buy, etc.

They destroy themselves, and find that their pathology might be very useful for the family.
"Mother you have to thank me. Because of my sickness you can experience how to cope with a sick person. So you have to thank me."

Strong sense of anger, completely self destructive, but obliging the system to take care of them.

Case: Patient, male, 27 years old, 35 kg!

Was sent by a colleague physiotherapist.

Worst disease Massimo has ever seen. Looked like coming from Mauthausen, almost unable to walk. Had been treated in hospital for 15 years without solution.

"Collagenosis" - no precise diagnosis. Sclerodermia, Raynaud, Myo- Joint-problems. St. p. amputation of fingers and toes. Stumps not healing, continuous use of antibiotics and cortisones. Infected ulcers.
Mouth full of Candida, lost several teeth, rest of teeth full of caries.

Before beginning secondary school, he wanted to become expert in music, then theatre and art, then programmer ... His father is butcher, his mother is helping in the store. 4-5 years playing around, theorizing and fantasising that the school is not good enough... then the parents forced him to work. When he started to touch the cold meat, he first got Raynaud's Disease, followed soon by his first gangrene.

Contact impossible, had seen lots of doctors without result, without expectations.

Raynaud worse and worse, sclerodermia going deeper- lungs, spleen, liver with fibrosis. In the beginning lot of pain in muscles and joints. Herpes zoster, red patches on the skin. Takes lots of Cortisone.

Strong headache from hypertension (RR 180/120) due to fibrosis. Blood pressure should not be lowered because of gangrene.

Lot of pain in extremities: cold, purple, ulcers, necrosis (less pain).

Ischemia was worse in summer that led to amputation of fingers and toes.

Antibodies increasing, thrombosis.

"Cannot open my mouth so easily. There is a persistent cough, never at night, mainly in company."

Fibrosis in lungs, enteritis, diarrhoea, food difficult to absorb > blueberry.
"The only thing I can digest is very heavy food, like meat with heavy sauce."

"There were psychosomatic problems in family, I was obliged to work with my father, then I was in a different butchery. Nobody understood me, when I had to wash clothes I started with the cough, they used some acids there."

"I do not like to stay with my family. I started to quarrel with my parents in primary school, when forced to work it went worse. I was lost with my mind, could not study, had to repeat twice a class in primary school."

"I want to study, to read, but the only book was the prophecy of Celestine. I enjoy different kinds of music, esp. heavy metal. More important is the kind of sound (aggressive) than the melody. It is the only way to discharge my anger, that I kept inside for years and that I could not solve. Just the music can help me."

"I had a dream: I wanted to fly to the jungle in Australia, but forgot my passport, was dropped in Italy and got sick"

"I am angry with myself, I was not able to do what I wanted, and with the persons around me. They are obstacles for me; they never helped me in my way and always pushed me where they wanted. I was not strong enough to do what I wanted; now I am obliged to continue like that. My problem is that I do not have a goal in my life."

First remedy: Hura brasiliensis – no effect

Second prescription: Sulfuricum acidum

In a short time stopped taking any remedy, started psychoanalysis, left Italy. His mother had to take him to a warm place at the seaside. She had to leave her work and went to the Canary Islands for some months. He told her every day how little she understood him and how badly his family had supported him. Back in Italy he started to do something for himself.

Follow-up after 4 years:

No infections any more, M. Raynaud much better, blood pressure needs. /100 diast, gained weight (about 10 kg!). Can breathe and walk without any difficulty.

Sulfuricum Acidum Rubrics:

Music ameliorates

Ailments from vexation

Emaciation

Extremities, ulcers, fingers

PICRICUM ACIDUM

Description

Pharmacopoiea: Common name: English: Trinitrophenol Picric acid;
French: Acide picrique;
German: Pikrinsäure

Picric acid or Trinitrophenol C_6H_2 $(NO_2)_{3OH}$ is one of the more dangerous chemicals used today. It is a flammable solid when mixed with more than 30% water (UN1344, class 4.1) and a class a high explosive with less than 30% water (UN0154, class 1.1D)

It is explosive but also highly shock, heat and friction sensitive. In fact, detonation with a speed and power superior to that of TNT can occur by a 2 kg weight falling on to solid picric acid from a height of 36 cm.

Picric acid is a derivative of phenol; it reacts with active metals (e.g. Ag, Pb, Ca, K) to form metal picrates, which are highly sensitive explosives.

Higher yields are obtained if chlorobenzene is used as a starting material instead of synthesizing by nitration of phenol. Picric acid is highly reactive with a wide variety of chemicals and extremely susceptible to the formation of picrate salts. Many of these salts are even more reactive and shock sensitive than the acid itself.

The pale yellow needles or crystals are odourless and have an intensely bitter taste. This bitter taste is known since ancient times and gives the origin of its name. Greek. *pikros*, πικροσ = "bitter".

It is soluble in most organic solvents, sparingly soluble in cold water; more soluble in hot water; soluble in alcohol; prepared by sulphonating phenol and then treating the reaction mixture with nitric acid. Contains not less than 99.0 percent of C6H3N3O7.

Wt. per ml.: 1.760 to 1.765.

Melting point: 121 to 123.

Water insoluble matter: Not more than 0.02 percent.

Caution: Explosive when dry, rapidly heated or by percussion. Handle with care. For safety in transportation, it is mixed with 10 to 15 percent water.

Traditional use

Picric acid is used primarily in the manufacture of explosives (matches and gunpowder).

In addition to its use in explosives, picric acid has been used as a yellow dye, as an antiseptic, and in the synthesis of chloropicrin, or nitrotrichloromethane, CCl_3NO_2, a powerful insecticide.

It is also present in many laboratories, for use as a chemical reagent. Water is added to picric acid to act as a desensitiser. The wet product is significantly less shock sensitive than the dry acid.

At the beginning of the 20th century it was used as an astringent, as disinfectant, also as an analgesic after burning.

Because of its poisonous character it is no longer used today. For the same reason it is now less used as a dye and explosive for military use.

Toxicology

Picric acid is toxic for our physical body (lethal dose 1 - 2g)

All routes of entry, skin and horny skin are irritated, they become yellow after long exposure. Picric acid is an allergen and produces toxic products on decomposition. Picric acid destroys the red cells and renal organs.

As an insecticide it corrodes the mucous membranes, and decomposes protein and the blood.

Neurotoxic (eyes, ears), ascending paralysis with cerebral activity.

Homeopathy

History and authority

Proved by Parisel in 1868; Allen: Enclop. Mat. Med., Vol.VII, 519; Hering: Guiding Symptoms, Vol.VIII. 437.

Preparation:

(a) Mother Tincture Q Drug Strength 1/100. Acidum Picricum, in crystalline powder 10g

Strong alcohol in sufficient quantity to make one thousand millilitres of the Mother Tincture (b) Potencies: 3x and higher with Dispensing Alcohol.

Themes and rubrics

The chief field for Acidum Picricum is the severe nervous exhaustion.
Mental work, reading and writing exhaust, can no longer be concentrated. It can proceed to a complete loss of energy and mental power.

Cannot maintain and sustain any structure

They do their best to keep all the parts together, they keep the family together. Need a rigid environment, often an overprotective family. Even if it is a terrible family, they are like a "container" for the unit (desire to be bandaged!)

Rubrics:
Prostration of mind
Vanishing of thoughts
The idea of marriage seems unendurable
 Lack of will power, as if they are mentally exhausted

Severe dependency

In the sense of strong restriction. They reduce their life to a minimum. Feel unable to do something that makes sense. See themselves as standing at the edge of the system. Feeling, he is a "failure" in his family and he could never cope with their expectations.

Cannot endure normal pressure

Lots of **rubrics** of inner pressure,
("There is something explosive inside myself, that I have to suppress, otherwise everything would be destroyed" – almost destroys himself – emaciation!)
Bursting, pressing sensation,
Sexual overload
Pressure has to be revealed, better when bandaged
Head, abdomen

A **Glonoin** - like headache indeed appears with picric acid nevertheless the vascular action is subordinate.

Headaches "up to bursting" begin in the Occiput and extend forward to the eyes: they are relieved by tightly binding the head and are worse from movement, from any effort, from dazzling light, from summer heat, in warm rooms, better in the fresh air and lying down. The pains also extend over the neck to the back along the vertebral column.

Congestion (theme of all acids)

Explosive substances often show symptoms of congestion, possibly to be seen as explosive feeling.

Feeling of heaviness

Hypertension

Desire for cold fresh air

Bipolarity (weakness - - - sexual overload)

Weakness in general

The spinal cord centres for the sexual functions are also especially involved

Sexual complaints

Suppressed sexual desire agg

Sexual weakness, with seminal emissions, spermatorrhea, states of irritation and priapism from spinal cord diseases and finally impotence.

(The nerve centres of the spinal cord are affected. Also the medulla, cerebellum and cerebrum)

Rubrics:

Male; EJACULATIONS, seminal discharge; premature, too quick (45) *Male; ERECTIONS, troublesome; continued (77) **Male; ERECTIONS, troublesome; strong (violent) (36) ***Male; POLLUTIONS, seminal emissions; night; every

Female, menses, pruritus vulvae, before

Female, menses dysmenorrhoea

Vertigo and ear noises (recalling those of ac.salicylicum and ac benz.)

Important relation to renal organs (toxicology!) / **urogenital system**

Rubrics:

Dribbling urination

Nocturnal urgency

Kidney and urinary passage in general, strangury is also observed in poisoning.

Sub acute nephritis with many renal elements and scanty, dark urine particularly in outstanding exhaustion.

Pain in gen : pressing

Back

Picricum acidum played a great role in older medicine for "spinal irritation": There is a burning and sensation of heat along the vertebra with extreme paralytic-like weakness in the back and in the legs, numbness

Sensations of tenseness in various places, particularly in the legs and feet. It is hard to keep the feet warm.

Partial hyperirritability syndrome like writer's cramps.

Case: Amintore is 62 years old

He comes to his appointment with his elder sister. They are a strange couple which seems to have come from a book from the turn of the century: their language, their body movements and what they say about what they do all day gives the impression of a couple of bigots who have not yet figured out we are at the end of the twentieth century. They live together and they never got married: the Lady comes across as the dominant one and during the visit she acts like an apprehensive and bossy mother in relationship to her child. Amintore takes it all without a fight, with a not so smart looking look and like a dog that has been beaten, I often have to intervene to let him speak. His sister decided he needed to be seen and she has decided to come to me because one of her friends, who are one of my patients, mentioned my name.

The woman begins:

"Ever since he was a little boy he has been confused. But I am not his mother and I cannot follow him around it's about time that he would stop being so needy also because I have already had to spend so much money with doctors and medicine and we are always at the same starting point. We have been going to doctors forever"

I ask Amintore what this is all about but his sister answers:

"He no loner sleeps at night and he doesn't let me sleep either because I can't sleep knowing that he is awake in the house, I don't know what he's up to and then he sleeps during the day instead of going shopping and I have to take care of all the housework by myself"

I insist asking the same question to Amintore and I motion to the lady to let him speak:

"I have been suffering from insomnia for years but until now I did OK with the various medicines I was taking, now they no longer have effect on me and I am very tired during the day, so much so I am unable to keep my eyes open, and then at night I can't fall asleep. I lay awake for hours looking at the ceiling and during the day I am unable to stand up, my eyes close and I have to sleep."

I ask Amintore what type of remedies he has tried in the past:

"I spent years in the house trying various cures, if I count all the months I spent being treated. I even had electroshock three times"

I ask him what type of problems he used to have and his sister intervenes: "I was losing a lot of weight and he never would eat we saw many doctors but he had some real internal problems and he would always get wasted and he almost lost his sight a long with his mind"

I motion to the Lady to let her brother talk:

"I remember they used to tell me I had satyriasis because I would have nightly losses and more than once I would really get thin and would be wiped out"

I ask for further explanations:

"I started wetting the bed when I was 12 and after a few years I went through months when it would happen even for a month in a row and I was not doing too well and I couldn't do anything, not even go to school. They had me do so many bromide treatments, the stuff they used to give to soldiers, and then in the end they shocked me, three times and then the problems went away."

The sister intervenes: "He is starting it all up over again and ever since he started to follow our doctor's new cures he is unable to sleep again, just like he used to do so many years ago which is why I decided to take him here right away to take care of him before he gets as bad as he was so many years ago that he looked like a corpse"

I ask Amintore what he used to do in the past:

"I worked as a phone operator for a few years in the city hall and then I retired with a disability pension"

I ask some more about his work "I have always been a simple person ever since I was in school. I was really shy and I was always afraid of making a mistake, even when I was a phone operator and I had to speak to people without seeing their face. When the office manager would call me I felt bad and I would sweat a lot even when I was a boy in boarding school I was unable to speak and when I was at the board and I really didn't do too well in school"

I ask him why he had to go to boarding school and the sister answers again:

"My poor parents sent him there because he just couldn't study. Our city had a very good religious boarding school and they sent him there because they said he really had no system, but even there it was a problem for my parents because he simply refused to study"

Amintore shyly intervenes:

"I couldn't study, I was always sick and I have never been able to remember things, I hated to read and to be in front of a book for hours on end and then the Salesians scared me to death with their punishments. They even made me read the same things one hundred times while kneeling on beans"

I decide not to push too much since I notice how the patient is feeling very em-barrassed and sullen, and furthermore I really don' t think the answers are very free and truthful especially in the presence of his sister the hag. As I am looking at the list of symptoms the Lady adds:

"Also tell him that you don't eat hardly anything and that you are always getting thinner, if you keep eating without cooking no wonder you are not able to digest anything!"

I ask Amintore for an explanation:

"I have never been able to eat cooked food, they used to scream at me also when I was little but it burns my stomach if I don't let the food cool down, I have to eat things that don't burn and drink things that don't burn otherwise I will ruin my stomach. I am simply unable to drink hot things I really like them much better if I add ice"

The sister intervenes once again:

"But not even all frozen, why should I cook if you are going to let it get cold"

Based on the symptoms listed in the medical materia I decide to prescribe PICRICUM ACIDUM 200K since it appears to be the remedy that matches the symptoms presented by the patient. A few days later the hag calls me back to complain that her brother is getting worse because his nocturnal emissions are much more frequent even if the sleeping patterns have improved. I try to calm the lady down but the task is quite a challenge. Three months later Amintore calls me to tell me he is calling while his sister went shopping and that he has been trying to reach me for a few days and that he is glad to get a hold of me. Amintore wants to know if he can take the remedy again without a prescription because he says he has been feeling much better and he has been sleeping well and feeling very well over all. I calm the patient down and I ask him if he would like to come back to see me without his sister. I feel he is tentative about it and I let him know I am willing to meet him when his sister is out of the house and a further tentative try on his part makes me understand that if we met it would be economically difficult for him and I assure him that the meeting would just be a control and that he would not have to pay anything. I therefore meet the patient on his own about a month after the first visit and I feel he is a lot less uptight and his general appearance is a lot less stupid looking.

He spontaneously reports:

"I really feel good. A lot better than I had for years. I sleep well now but I wanted to talk with you by myself because I was embarrassed in front of my sister. I understand now that you are not a typical doctor and I trust you"

I ask him to explain what he means about feeling better:

"I feel stronger and less confused I sleep well now and I don't think it is only because of the medicine I am thinking that I cannot handle my sister anymore and that perhaps even she can help me. I had trouble sleeping because I also knew what could happen during sleep, even years ago I was afraid of sleep because I was afraid of all those losses. As time went by it became a habit and I didn't sleep any more during the night"

I ask Amintore if he remembers any dreams:

"I don't dream about women, many times I ejaculate without any excitement at all and I find myself all wet and if I get up to wash myself I end up getting wet again whereas if I leave it like it is it is easier that it may not happen again"

I underline I was not just interested in erotic dreams:

"I often dream about a river that is overflowing and that I am throwing paper boats in it but I don't know if it is a dream or a memory from when I was little, we used to live near the Po River"

I ask about his eating habits:

"I really don't pay much attention to it, as long as it isn't hot I eat everything in sight but I feel hot food all the way down my oesophagus, whereas cold food makes my insides feel good and I feel better"

I ask him if he remembers anything from the times he was hospitalised:

"I remember all the days spent in there, but I changed places often until they shocked me. I did all right there, I went there willingly because I felt protected and because they told me I would get rid of that disease. It was really embarrassing to always have an erection without any external excitement and to loose so much it seemed as if it would never end. I have never understood where all that stuff came from, even the doctors where amazed at how much semen came out, where did it all get into me"

I ask him if he remembers anything about his days in the boarding school:

"I was very timid and then I really didn't understand anything they were trying to teach me. My parents spent a lot of money to give me a good education but I was never able to repay them it was something stronger than myself but if I really put myself in front of a book it felt as if I were in front of somebody I didn't know, somebody who was not possible to get to know."

I ask something about his relationship with his sister:

"She runs my life_ she stays right after me. I have always lived with the family and she thinks about everything, also about my retirement. I had some troubles in that regard I have no money because my sister takes care of all the books, like all the other stuff around the house."

I ask him if he wants to tell me something about his relationship with women:

"I am a very practicing catholic, what can I say I have been with a prostitute a few times but it was really too much for me. Women are not an important aspect of my life."

I ask him to tell me what's important in his life:

"Health and God, if you don't have these things nothing else really matters"

I prescribe PICRICUM ACIDUM 1000 and we agree to meet next whenever possible. Within six months I receive a phone call from Amintore who is very happy about how he is feeling also because his nocturnal emissions have subsided but he is starting to have some insomnia again. After a placebo, which had no effect whatsoever, I prescribe 10M. Six months go by and Amintore is back again after making an appointment like anybody else.

"I have changed late but at least I have changed. I went to live with a friend and I left my sister. I couldn't take it anymore I talked about this for a long time with my spiritual father who told me that if I wanted live my life like this I should.

But I don't want to live by myself, I can't after sixty years but I know I can't live with my sister any more even if that means I have to live on my own. I cannot also ruin the last years of my life, but it really upset her and she is upset with you because she says that after your treatment I got these ideas and that now I am unthankful to her after all these years."

I ask him about his sleep:

"I sleep now whenever I want to and when I am tired I sleep well. I eat whenever I feel like it and I even eat spaghetti with ice which I ate at the Unita' festival. I had them teach me the Japanese recipe. I have had no more nocturnal emissions and I feel much stronger and more in control of myself. I also retired on my own and in the evenings I play cards with my friend never for money I have any vices. The only vice I really have are romance novels, I found a collection of them in the newspaper stand and I avidly read them without much effort and I feel very satisfied"

Over several years Amintore is doing fine and he is still living with his friend. I have occasionally prescribed the remedy in various dilutions during a few flu episodes and the remedy has worked up until now.

HYDROCYANICUM ACIDUM

Description

HCN being a colourless liquid with a smell of bitter almonds has a certain similarity to water with which it easily combines. Its melting point is minus 13,24° C and its boiling point is 25,7°C. HCN, whether liquid or gaseous, is extremely toxic. It hampers oxygenation of haemoglobin in red blood cells.

Sources

Some plants' seeds contain a considerable amount of cyanogene glycosides (e.g. bitter almond, peach, apricot, cherry, plum), which may be transformed into hydrocyanic acid under suitable conditions. HCN contained in 60 bitter almonds is lethal for adults, for children 5-10 suffice. Fruit juice or jam may contain HCN if their stones are smashed during the production process. In spite of this dangerous fact, they are purposely smashed in order to ameliorate taste.

The Lima Bean may also contain HCN, its source being "Linamarin". It was possible to reduce Linamarin in the cultivated white form, whereas the colored wild form still contains a high quantity.

Maniok (=Cassava), a basic aliment for more than 400 million people in the Third World, contains an alarmingly high concentration of HCN. Already the consumption of 200 to 500 grams of fresh bulb may be fatal. This is why only detoxicated bulbs may be used in aliments. In principle, this is quite a simple process: the bulbs are shred or pulverized, thus destroying the plant cells, resulting in an enzymatic separation of HCN, which evaporates during the following dehydration process. As a rule, Maniok flour resulting from this procedure can be used as nourishment at no risk.

Improper detoxication may cause chronic HCN-intoxication. Whereas acute poisoning is mainly caused by HCN itself, chronic disease is often caused by its metabolites. The constant catabolism of hydrocyanic acid by the enzyme Rhodanase in human organism leads to a chronic high blood concentration of Rhodanid. This interferes with the uptake of Iodine in the thyroid gland, resulting in the typical deficiency symptoms, such as struma and cretinism.

HCN may as well damage the nervous system. Certain kinds of diabetes may be associated.

Traditional and nowadays use

In ancient Egypt priests prepared an infusion of peach stones, the so-called "drink of silence", leading to death.

Dioskurides' scriptures, kept in the museum of Louvre, say "Don't mention the name of JAO on penalty of peach".

Umberto Ecco "In the name of the rose": pages marked with HCN lead to intoxication when turning the page.

As "Prussic Acid" used as pesticide. Since 1887 used as an insecticide against shild-lice on orange-plantation.

Cyanide caustic solutions were used to dissolve gold and silver.

During the 2nd World War the SS – in their extermination camps - used the hydro-cyanic acid compound "Cyclone B" which evaporated by body temperature and led to death from suffocation within a very short time.

Cyanic acid (Y=O) as well as Thiocyanic Acid (Y=S) can be generated *in situ* by dissolving potassium cyanate or potassium thiocyanate in acetic acid or formic acid. Thus equilibrium between two tautomeric forms of the according acid is established, providing cyanic or thiocyanic acid – the presumed active species in the CYCLOADDITION REACTION to hydrazones.

Cyanide wastewater treatment
Cyanide wastewater is treated according to the alkaline-chlorine oxidation method; that is to say, cyanides are first changed into cyanic acid and then decomposed into carbon dioxide gas and nitrogen gas. Metals in cyanide wastewater are separated by sedimentation as metal hydroxide. Supernatant liquor is discharged out of the plant. Sedimented sludge is dehydrated and a subcontractor carries out disposal.

Toxicology

Larger amounts of HCN lead to difficult respiration, dilation of pupils, cramps and to death from suffocation within a few seconds.

As human beings as well as mammals possess a well-functioning decontamination system for HCN, the lethal dose is relatively high: adults 50 mg free HCN/day. Little doses of HCN that may be found in a large number of aliments cause no health problem whatsoever. 20 to 30 mg HCN may easily be transformed per day by the adult liver through the enzyme Rhodanase into non-toxic Rhodanid, excreted by urine.

The toxic potential of HCN is due to the ability to build stable complexes with metal-ions, thus blocking a number of important enzymes, among others cytochromes responsible for vesicular breathing. This leads to dying of cells.

Sensitive insects: flies, butterflies.

Relatively resistant: cockroaches, mealworms.

Poisoning is severe and fast! If survived, no persisting damage remains.

Detoxication with Sulphur – forms thiocyanide.

Homeopathy

Cramps (more than in other acids) children, newborns: opisthotonus (body stiffens and is thrown back with cyanosis), hysteric and epileptic, trismus, clenched teeth, impulse to bite.

Larynx, Trachea

Respiration

Cough

Strong despair

Fear of being run over, by something that is stronger than you, of public places, of a crowd, crossing streets, waterish element, that is running over him. Idea of something is moving around you (then even the sun could be a danger)

Vertigo
Waves, objects are turning

High sense of duty
Feeling to have a huge task in front of him with sensation of being small and weak.

Reaction: sudden acting out, self-destructive, injuring themselves, tendency to mutilate his body.

Case: Lady, 58 yrs. old

Dressed in a strange way, giving a lot of attention to her appearance, too much perfume, red stockings, masculine way. Problems to express herself – very talkative, but giving the impression of not having enough time to tell everything.

MM could already hear her coughing in the waiting room in a very loud and convulsive way.

Her husband had passed away 2 years ago; she was living with her two sons now. When she moved into the house, there were 4 generations living there. Her father-in-law was a disabled soldier; two family members were suffering from cancer with metastasis in the bones. She was always taking care of them, she knew every hospital around. The mother-in-law, suffering from breast-cancer she, had been doing everything for her husband, always hiding her own disease. Her husband had started his own enterprise with the help of investors, who only took profit of the company without working themselves. He had his own trade-mark in ceramics. When he became sick, the partnership turned out to be quite difficult, since they were depending on his manpower. So the patient took over the enterprise, she purchased the whole company. She had a very good relation-ship with her husband for 40 years and since his death she felt an enormous emptiness inside.

She was suffering from back pains, and had already received various therapies. Many years ago, when bathing in the sea, a huge wave caused perforation of her tympanum, a fact she realized only years later. 10 years ago, during the operation for a tympanoplastic, a middle ear bone was broken and the nerve was cut. Since that time there was a chronic discharge from the ear, which had to be cleaned regularly. Hearing was impaired hence and she was suffering from a metallic taste constantly.

Her dentist, who treated her for malocclusion, sent her. She was grinding teeth during sleep so severely that her ceramic crowns were broken.

She had a craving for sweets and especially chocolate.

There were many injuries in the past. She described her skiing attempts as a "massacre". She called it "hanging myself" when she talked about relaxing her vertebral column, thus using rather destroying expressions.

Further complaints were: vertigo with nausea, waking during the night with cervical pains.

Awful fear of water since she was a child (only shower possible, no bath!).

At the age of 23 she had hepatitis.

When her father died at the age of 58, she felt guilty for not having been able to take care of him in a better way and she fell into a deep depression. At that time she promised herself to never get a depression again. So now, she was fighting against it with chocolate, and kept hiding her suffering from her family. "A man always needs the company of a woman who does not create any problems!"

Shortly before her husband had passed away, he apologized. Hence she was sleepless from intruding thoughts.

The main symptoms of her depression were: indifference to everybody, apathy, watching herself in the mirror and scratching her face, tearing nails and cuticle, plucking her eyebrows.

There was asthma in childhood. For more than 30 years she had been suffering from a suffocating cough (she could only stop coughing when she was not able to breath anymore). She used to sleep with oxygen every night.

Parturitions as well as menses had been very painful.

Therapy: Hydr. -Ac. Q1 for 3 days (later Q3 for some days)
Next day painful abscess in the mouth, opened by the dentist and treated with antibiotics. She almost finished homeopathic treatment.

Sleep was improving.
Dream: her father calls her for help, but as she is lying on her healthy ear, she cannot hear him. (Hydrocyanic Acidum often dreams about being asked for help with impossibility to help).
The chronic cough improved a lot – no need for oxygen any more.
As she had always loved the seaside, she finally moved to her house in Florida, where she never could sleep in former times due to her hydrophobia. So she left her family to live on her own "It's my turn now."

INDEX